HORMONE

FIGHTING HORMONE IMBALANCE

The Keto Way To Fight Hormone Imbalance, Acne, and Indigestion With Low Carb, Low Sugar, and A Proven Meal Plan & Workout Plan

DARIO MONTES

Table of Contents

PART I

Hormone Diet

Are you worried that your hormones are not at their optimal levels? Here is a diet that will solve your problems.

Chapter 1: Health Benefits of the Hormone Diet

When it comes to getting healthy through weight loss, there's never any shortage of fitness crazes and diets that claim to have the secret to easy and sustainable weight loss. One of the latest diet plans that have come into the spotlight is the hormone diet, which claims that people often struggle to lose weight because of their hormones.

A hormone diet is a 3-step process that spans over six weeks and is designed to synchronize your hormones and promote a healthy body through detoxification, nutritional supplements, exercise, and diet. The diet controls what you eat and informs you about the correct time to eat to ensure maximum benefits to your hormones. Many books have been written on this topic with supporters of the diet assuring people that they can lose weight quickly and significantly through diet and exercise and reset or manipulate their hormones. Although the diet has a few variations, the central idea around each is that correcting the body's perceived hormonal imbalances is the key to losing weight.

The most important benefit of a hormone diet is that it takes a solid stance on improving overall health through weight loss and promoting regular exercise as well as natural, nutritious foods. Apart from that, it also focuses on adequate sleep, stress management, emotional health, and other healthy lifestyle habits that are all essential components that people should follow, whether it's a part of a diet or not. Including a water diet, it aims towards losing about twelve pounds in the 1st phase and 2 pounds a week after that.

Hormones have an essential role in the body's everyday processes, like helping bones grow, digesting food, etc. They act as "chemical messengers," instructing the cells to perform specific actions and are transported around the body through the bloodstream.

One of the very important food items to be included in the hormone diet is salmon. Salmon is rich in omega-3 fatty acids, Docosahexaenoic acid, and Eicosapentaenoic acid (EPA). It is rich in selenium too. These help to lower your blood pressure and also reduce the level of unhealthy cholesterol in the blood. These make you less prone to heart diseases. Salmon is a rich source of healthy fat. If consumed in sufficient amounts, it provides you energy and helps you get rid of unwanted body fat. Salmon is well-known for giving fantastic weight loss results as it has less saturated fat, unlike other protein sources. Salmon is packed with vitamins like vitamin-k, E, D, and A. These are extremely helpful for your eyes, bone joints, etc. These vitamins are also good for your brain, regulation of metabolic balance, and repairing your muscles. Salmon's vitamins and omega-3 fatty acids are amazing for sharpening your mind. It also improves your memory retention power. If you consume salmon, you are less likely to develop dementia or mental dis-functions. Salmon has anti-inflammatory properties and is low in omega-6 fatty acid content (which is pro-inflammatory in nature and is present in a huge amount in the modern diet). It promotes healthy skin and gives you radiant and glowing skin. It is good for the winter because it helps you to stay warm. It also provides lubrication to your joints because of the abundant presence of essential minerals and fatty acids in it. Apart from this, some other things to include in your diet are arugula, kale, ginger, avocado, carrots, and so on.

There are almost sixteen hormones that can influence weight. For example, the hormone leptin produced by your fat cells is considered a "satiety hormone," which makes you feel full by reducing your appetite. As a signaling hormone, it communicates with the part of your brain (hypothalamus) that controls food intake and appetite. Leptin informs the brain when there is enough fat in storage, and extra fat is not required. This helps prevent overeating. Individuals who are obese or overweight generally have very high levels of leptin in their blood. Research shows that the level of leptin in obese individuals was almost four times higher than that in individuals with normal weight.

Studies have found that fat hormones like leptin and adiponectin can promote long-term weight loss by reducing appetite and increasing metabolism. It is believed that both these fat hormones follow the same pathway in the brain to manage blood sugar (glucose) and body weight (Robert V. Considine, 1996).

Simply put, the hormone diet works by helping to create a calorie deficit through better nutritional habits and exercise, which ultimately results in weight loss. It's also essential to consult a doctor before following this detox diet or consuming any dietary supplements.

Chapter 2: Hormone-Rebalancing Smoothies

Estrogen Detox Smoothie

Total Prep & Cooking Time: 5 minutes

Yields: One glass

Nutrition Facts: Calories: 312 | Carbs: 47.9g | Protein: 18.6g | Fat: 8.5g | Fiber: 3g

Ingredients:

- Half a cup of hemp seeds
- Two kiwis (medium-sized)
- A quarter each of
  - Avocado (medium-sized)
  - Cucumber (medium-sized)
- Half a unit each of
  - Lemon (squeezed freshly)
  - Green apple
- One celery (medium-sized)
- A quarter cup of cilantro
- Two tbsps. of chis seeds
- Two cups of water (filtered)
- One tsp. of cacao nibs
- One tbsp. of coconut oil

Method:

1. Blend the ingredients all together to form a smoothie at high speed. The thickness can be adjusted according to your preference by adding more water to the mixture.

2. Serve and enjoy.

Dopamine Delight Smoothie

Total Prep Time: 10 minutes

Yields: One serving

Nutrition Facts: Calories: 383 | Carbs: 31g | Protein: 24g | Fat: 18.g | Fiber: 3g

Ingredients:

- Half a teaspoon of cinnamon (ground)
- Half a cup of peeled banana (the bananas must be frozen)
- One organic espresso, double shot (measuring half a cup)
- One tablespoon of chia seeds
- A three-fourth cup of soy milk (plain or vanilla-flavored)
- Protein powder, a serving (from the whey with the flavor of vanilla)

Method:

1. Fill in the bowl of your blender with all the ingredients (from the section of ingredients) except the whey protein powder and then proceed by switching to a high-speed blending option. Make sure it acquires a smooth consistency and then pour it out.

2. Now you may add the protein powder and give it another shot of blend until the whole things get incorporated, a bit of the goat cheese (already crumbled).

Breakfast Smoothie Bowl

Total Prep Time: 10 minutes

Yields: 2 servings

Nutrition Facts: Calories: 290 | Carbs: 53g | Protein: 6g | Fat: 8g | Fiber: 9g

Ingredients:

- One cup of thoroughly rinsed blueberries (fresh and ripe)
- A sundry of nuts and fruits for garnishing, which includes – strawberries, bananas (thinly sliced), peanuts (Spanish), kiwi (chopped), segments of tangerine, and raspberries.
- One cup of Greek yogurt

For the preparation of honey flax granola,

- Two tablespoons each of
  o Flaxseeds
  o Vegetable oil
- Oats (old-fashioned), approximately a cup
- One tablespoon of honey

Method:

1. Set your oven at a temperature of 350 degrees F.

2. Preparation of the smoothie: collect the diverse types of berries, wash them thoroughly, and then put them in the blender and turn it on. Make an even mixture out of it. Add some amount of the yogurt and blend it again to form a smooth texture.

3. For preparing the granola: Take a small-sized bowl and then drizzle a few drops oil in it. Then add the oats, flax, and honey to the oil, one by one, and mix it well. You are required to toss the bowl thoroughly to get the mixture well-coated with the poured oil. After you are done, place the oats mixture in a baking sheet evenly. Bake it for about twenty minutes. This mark will be enough to give the oats a beautiful tinge of golden brown. Allow it to cool.

4. Now you will require a shallow bowl to spoon in some yogurt, and this will be the first layer. Form a second layer with the various fruits and nuts and finally for the third layer, top with the granola.

5. Enjoy.

Notes:

*   *Using frozen nuts and fruits in a warm-weather will get much to your relief.*

*   *For a vegan smoothie bowl, sub the yogurt with coconut or almond yogurt.*

*   *Give the pan a few strokes while baking the oats.*

Blueberry Detox Smoothie

Total Prep Time: Ten minutes

Yields: One serving

Nutrition Facts: Calories: 326 | Carbs: 65g | Protein: 4g | Fat: 8g | Fiber: 9g

Ingredients:

- One cup of wild blueberries (frozen)
- One banana (sliced into several pieces) frozen
- Orange juice (approximately half a cup)
- Cilantro leaves, fresh (approximately a measuring a small handful size)
- A quarter of an entire avocado
- A quarter cup of water

Method:

1. Add cilantro, avocado, water, blueberries, banana, and orange juice in the blender and then process.

2. Make the ingredients integrated so well that they become smooth in their consistency.

Notes: *It is recommended that you add the potent herb, cilantro, or parsley in a small amount when consuming this smoothie for the first time, as it might trigger a mild headache. If you do not get a headache, you may add a bit more of the cilantro leaves.*

Maca Mango Smoothie

Total Prep & Cooking Time: 2 minutes

Yields: 2 servings

Nutrition Facts: Calories: 53 | Carbs: 13g | Protein: 1g | Fat: 3g | Fiber: 1.5g

Ingredients:

- One and a half cups each of
  - Fresh mango
  - Frozen mango
- One tablespoon each of
  - Ground flaxseed
  - Nut butter
- One teaspoon of ground turmeric
- Two teaspoons of maca root powder
- Three-quarter cups of nut milk
- One frozen banana

Method:

1. Blend all the ingredients together to get a smooth mixture.

2. Adjust consistency by adding nut milk.

3. Once done, divide into two glasses and enjoy!

Pituitary Relief Smoothie

Total Prep & Cooking Time: 5 minutes

Yields: 2 servings

Nutrition Facts: Calories: 174 | Carbs: 18.3g | Protein: 9.7g | Fat: 8.3g | Fiber: 14.4g

Ingredients:

- One teaspoon of coconut oil
- One fresh or frozen ripe banana
- One tablespoon of raw sesame seeds
- Two teaspoons each of
  o Chia seeds
  o Raw Maca powder
  o Raw Spirulina
- Two cups of water
- Two tablespoons of hulled hemp seeds

Method:

1. You have to use a blender to process this smoothie. Add the hulled hemp seeds, sesame seeds, and water in the blender and process them. Do it at high speed, and it will only require a minute. This will give you raw-milk like texture.

2. Then, add the following ingredients into it – coconut oil, banana, chia seeds, Maca, and Spirulina, and process the ingredients once again but this time on medium speed for another minute or so. Everything will become well incorporated.

3. You have to drink this smoothie on an empty stomach.

Notes: *In order to make the smoothie rich in antioxidants, you can add some fresh fruits like blueberries, kiwi, and raspberries.*

Chapter 2: Easy Breakfast Recipes

Scrambled Eggs With Feta and Tomatoes

Total Prep & Cooking Time: 10 minutes

Yields: One Plate

Nutrition Facts: Calories: 421 | Carbs: 8.6g | Protein: 20.3g | Fat: 35.1g | Fiber: 1.6g

Ingredients:

- One tbsp. each of
    - o Olive oil (extra virgin)
    - o Freshly chopped parsley, basil, dill or chives
- Half a cup of cherry tomatoes (each tomato sliced into half)
- Two ounces of crumbled feta cheese (approximately a quarter cup)
- Two eggs are beaten
- Two tbsp. of onion (diced)
- To taste:
    - o Black pepper
    - o Kosher salt

Method:

1. Keep the beaten eggs in a small-sized bowl and then season it with a pinch of pepper and salt. Set the bowl aside.

2. Use a nonstick skillet to proceed with the cooking. Pour two tbsp. of olive oil. Then add the diced onions. Stir over moderate heat and cook until softened. Make sure that the onions do not look brown. This process should get done by a minute.

3. Add half a cup of tomatoes to skillet and then continue to mix for about two minutes.

4. Now you may add the eggs. Using a spatula, gather the beaten eggs to the center by moving spatula all over the skillet.

5. The eggs will take an additional minute to get cooked. So after that mark, add the parsley or other herbs (if preferred) and feta cheese. Keep the eggs underdone as they will get cooked completely after they are served in the plate itself (from the residual heat). Therefore, cook the entire thing in the skillet for 30 seconds only.

6. Take a serving plate and transfer the eggs to it. Top with some sprinkled parsley and feta cheese, drizzled with some oil, and seasoned with some pepper and salt. These additions are optional and may vary as per your desire.

Smashed Avo and Quinoa

Total Prep & Cooking Time: 15 minutes

Yields: Six bowls

Nutrition Facts: Calories: 492 | Carbs: 67g | Protein: 15g | Fat: 20g | Fiber: 13g

Ingredients:

- One avocado skinned, cut into half, and then pitted
- A handful of cilantro or coriander
- Half a lemon (juiced)
- A quarter red onion (diced finely)
- One-eighth teaspoon of cayenne pepper
- To taste: Sea salt

For the Greens,

- One handful of kale
- One handful of soft herbs (basil, parsley or mint)
- One handful of chard or spinach
- For frying: butter or coconut oil

Serve with,

- One cup of quinoa (cooked)

Method:

1. You will require a frying pan to get this done. To it, add the coconut oil or butter (whichever you prefer) and add the greens. Toss them carefully and then sauté over moderate heat. Stop when they become soft.

2. Mix the onion, cayenne, avocado, cilantro, salt, lemon, and pepper to a bowl and mix them completely. The pepper and salt must be added according to the taste.

3. Add cooked quinoa to the tossed greens and heat altogether over low heat.

4. Take a serving plate and place the quinoa mixture and greens to it. Crown the whole thing with smashed avocado and then serve.

Hormone Balancing Granola

Total Prep & Cooking Time: 35 minutes

Yields: 8 servings

Nutrition Facts: Calories: 360 | Carbs: 19.8g | Protein: 5.1g | Fat: 28.8g | Fiber: 5.8g

Ingredients:

- One-third cup each of
  - Flaxseed meal
  - Pumpkin seeds
  - Seedless raisins
- Two teaspoons of cinnamon
- One teaspoon of vanilla extract
- Four tablespoons of maple syrup
- Five tablespoons of melted coconut oil
- A quarter cup of unsweetened coconut flakes
- Two-thirds cup each of
  - Chopped pecans
  - Chopped brazil nuts
- Two tablespoons of ground chia seeds

Method:

1. Set the temperature of the oven to 180 degrees F and preheat.

2. In a food processor, chop the pecans and the Brazil nuts. Then, mix these chopped nuts with coconut flakes, seeds, and other nuts present in the list of ingredients.

3. Add maple syrup, coconut oil, cinnamon, and vanilla extract in a separate bowl and combine well.

4. Now, take the wet ingredients and pour them into the dry ingredients. Mix thoroughly so that everything has become coated properly.

5. Place the prepared mixture in the oven for half an hour and cook.

6. Once done, cut into pieces and serve.

Chapter 3: Healthy Lunch Recipes

Easy Shakshuka

Total Prep & Cooking Time: 30 minutes

Yields: Six servings

Nutrition Facts: Calories: 154 | Carbs: 4.1g | Protein: 9g | Fat: 7.8g | Fiber: 0g

Ingredients:

- Olive oil (extra virgin)
- Two chopped green peppers
- One teaspoon each of
  - Paprika (sweet)
  - Coriander (ground)
- A pinch of red pepper (flakes)
- Half a cup of tomato sauce
- A quarter cup each of
  - Mint leaves (freshly chopped)
  - Parsley leaves (chopped freshly)
- One yellow onion, large-sized (chopped)
- Two cloves of garlic, chopped
- Half a teaspoon of cumin (ground)
- Six cups of chopped tomatoes (Vine-ripe)
- Six large-sized eggs
- To taste: Pepper and salt

Method:

1. You will require a large-sized skillet (made of cast iron). Pour three tablespoons of oil and heat it. After bringing the oil to boil, add the peppers, spices, onions, garlic, pepper, and salt. Stir time to time to cook the veggies for five minutes until they become softened.

2. After the vegetables become soft, add the chopped tomatoes and then tomato sauce. Cover the skillet and simmer for an additional fifteen minutes.

3. Now, you may remove the lid from the pan and then cook a touch more to thicken the consistency. At this point, you may adjust the taste.

4. Make six cavities within the tomato mixture and crack one egg each inside the cavities.

5. Cover the skillet after reducing the heat and allow it to cook so that the eggs settle into the cavities.

6. Keep track of the time and accordingly uncover the skillet and then add mint and parsley. Season with more black and red pepper according to your desire. Serve them warm with the sort of bread you wish.

Ginger Chicken

Total Prep & Cooking Time: 50 minutes

Yields: Six Servings

Nutrition Facts: Calories: 310 | Carbs: 6g | Protein: 37g | Fat: 16g | Fiber: 1g

Ingredients:

- A one-kilogram pack of chicken thighs (skinless and boneless)
- Four cloves of garlic (chopped finely)
- A fifteen-gram pack of coriander (fresh and chopped)
- Two tablespoons of sunflower oil
- One teaspoon each of
  - Turmeric (ground)
  - Chili powder (mild)
- A four hundred milliliter can of coconut milk (reduced-fat)
- One cube of chicken stock
- One ginger properly peeled and chopped finely (it should be of the size of a thumb)
- One lime, juiced
- Two medium-sized onions
- One red chili, sliced and the seeds removed (fresh)

Method:

1. Make the chicken thighs into three large chunks and marinate them with chili powder, garlic, coriander (half of the entire amount), ginger, oil (one tbsp.), and lime juice. Cover the bowl after stirring them well and then store it in the fridge until oven-ready.

2. Marinade the chicken and keep overnight for better flavor.

3. Chop the onions finely (it is going to be the simplest for preparing the curry) before dropping them into the food processor. Pour oil into the frying pan (large-sized) and heat it. Then add chopped onions and stir them thoroughly for eight minutes until the pieces become soft. Then pour the turmeric powder and stir for an additional minute.

4. Now add the chicken mixture and cook on high heat until you notice a change in its color. Pour the chicken stock, chili, and coconut milk and after covering the pan simmer for another twenty minutes. Sprinkle the left-over coriander leaves and then serve hot.

5. Enjoy.

Carrot and Miso Soup

Total Prep & Cooking Time: 1 hour

Yields: Four bowls of soup

Nutrition Facts: Calories: 76 | Carbs: 8.76g | Protein: 4.83g | Fat: 2.44g | Fiber: 1.5g

Ingredients:

- Two tbsps. of oil
- Garlic, minced (four cloves)
- One inch of garlic (grated)
- Three tbsps. of miso paste (white)
- One diced onion
- One pound of carrot (sliced thinly)
- Four cups of vegetable stock
- To taste: Pepper and Salt

For garnishing,

- Two scallions (sliced thinly)
- Chili pepper (seven spices)
- One nori roasted (make thin slivers)
- Sesame oil

Method:

1. Using a soup pot will be convenient to proceed with. Pour oil in a pot and then heat over a high flame. Now you may put garlic, carrot, and onion and sauté them thoroughly. Cook for about ten minutes so that the onions turn translucent.

2. Then add the ginger and vegetable stock. Mix them well and cook all together. Put the flame to simmer. Cover the pot while cooking to make the carrot tender. This will take another thirty minutes.

3. Put off the flame and puree the soup with the help of an immersion blender.

4. Use a small-sized bowl to whisk together a spoonful of the soup and the white miso paste. Stir until the paste dissolve and pour the mixture back to the pot.

5. Add pepper and salt if required.

6. Divide the soup among four bowls and enrich its feel by adding scallions, sesame oil, seven spices, and nori.

Arugula Salad

Total Prep & Cooking Time: 1 hour 10 minutes

Yields: Two bowls of salad

Nutrition Facts: Calories: 336.8 | Carbs: 30.6g | Protein: 7.7g | Fat: 22.2g | Fiber: 7.3g

Ingredients:

For the salad,

- Two medium-sized beets (boiled or roasted for about an hour), skinned and sliced into pieces that can easily be bitten
- Four tablespoons of goat cheese
- Approximately 2.5 oz. of baby arugula (fresh)
- A quarter cup of walnuts (chopped roughly before toasting)

For the dressing,

- Three tablespoons of olive oil (extra virgin)
- A quarter tsp. each of
  o Mustard powder (dried)
  o Pepper
- Half a tsp. each of
  o Salt
  o Sugar

- One and a half tablespoons of lemon juice

Method:

1. For preparing the vinaigrette, place all the ingredients (listed in the dressing ingredients section) in a jar and then shake them to emulsify. At this stage, before starting with the process of emulsification, you may add or remove the ingredients as per your liking.

2. Get the salad assembled (again depending upon the taste you want to give it), add a fistful of arugula leaves, place some chopped beets (after they have been cooked), and finally the toasted walnuts (already chopped).

3. Drizzle vinaigrette over the salad and enjoy.

Notes:

- *Coat the beets with oil (olive), roll them up in an aluminum foil, and then roast the beets at a temperature of 400 degrees F.*

- *And for boiling the beets, immerse them in water after transferring to a pot and simmer them for 45 minutes.*

Kale Soup

Total Prep & Cooking Time: 55 minutes

Yields: 8 servings

Nutrition Facts: Calories: 277.3 | Carbs: 50.9g | Protein: 9.6g | Fat: 4.5g | Fiber: 10.3g

Ingredients:

- Two tbsps. of dried parsley
- One tbsp. of Italian seasoning
- Salt and pepper
- Thirty oz. of drained cannellini beans
- Six peeled and cubed white potatoes
- Fifteen ounces of diced tomatoes
- Six vegetable Bouillon cubes
- Eight cups of water
- One bunch of kale (with chopped leaves and stems removed)
- Two tbsps. of chopped garlic
- One chopped yellow onion
- Two tbsps. of olive oil

Method:

1. At first, take a large soup pot, add in some olive oil, and heat it.

2. Add garlic and onion. Cook them until soft.

3. Then stir in the kale and cook for about two minutes, until wilted.

4. Pour the water and add the beans, potatoes, tomatoes, vegetable bouillon, parsley, and the Italian seasoning.

5. On medium heat, simmer the soup for about twenty-five minutes, until the potatoes are cooked through.

6. Finally, do the seasoning with salt and pepper according to your taste.

Roasted Sardines

Total Prep & Cooking Time: 25 minutes

Yields: 4 servings

Nutrition Facts: Calories: 418 | Carbs: 2.6g | Protein: 41g | Fat: 27.2g | Fiber: 0.8g

Ingredients:

- 3.5 oz. of cherry tomatoes (cut them in halves)
- One medium-sized red onion (chopped finely)
- Two tablespoons each of
    - Chopped parsley
    - Extra-virgin olive oil
- One clove of garlic (halved)
- Eight units of fresh sardines (gutted and cleaned, heads should be cleaned)
- A quarter teaspoon of chili flakes
- One teaspoon of toasted cumin seeds
- Half a lemon (zested and juiced)

Method:

1. Set the temperature of the oven to 180 degrees C and preheat. Take a roasting tray and grease it lightly.

2. Take a bowl and add the tomatoes and onions in it. Add the lemon juice too and toss the veggies in the lemon juice. Now, add the zest, olive oil, chili, cumin, garlic, and parsley and toss everything once again.

3. Use pepper and salt to season the mixture. The cavity of the sardines has to be filled. Use some of the tomato and onion mixture for this purpose. Once done, place the sardines on the prepared roasting tray. Take the remaining mixture and scatter it over the sardines.

4. Roast the sardines for about 10-15 minutes, and by the end of this, they should be cooked thoroughly.

5. Serve and enjoy!

Chapter 4: Tasty Dinner Recipes

Rosemary Chicken

Total Prep & Cooking Time: 50 minutes

Yields: 4 servings

Nutrition Facts: Calories: 232 | Carbs: 3.9g | Protein: 26.7g | Fat: 11.6g | Fiber: 0.3g

Ingredients:

- Four chicken breast halves (skinless and boneless)
- One-eighth tsp. kosher salt
- One-fourth tsp. ground black pepper
- One and a half tbsps. of lemon juice
- One and a half tbsps. of Dijon mustard
- Two tbsps. of freshly minced rosemary
- Three tbsps. of olive oil
- Eight minced garlic cloves

Method:

1. At first, preheat a grill to medium-high heat. The grate needs to be lightly oiled.

2. Take a bowl and add lemon juice, mustard, rosemary, olive oil, garlic, salt, and ground black pepper. Whisk them together.

3. Take a resealable plastic bag and place the chicken breasts in it. Over the chicken, pour the garlic mixture (reserve one-eighth cup of it).

4. Seal the bag and start massaging the marinade gently into the chicken. Allow it to stand for about thirty minutes at room temperature.

5. Then on the preheated grill, place the chicken and cook for about four minutes.

6. Flip the chicken and baste it with the marinade reserved and then cook for about five minutes, until thoroughly cooked.

Finally, cover it with a foil and allow it to rest for about 2 minutes before you serve them.

Corned Beef and Cabbage

Total Prep & Cooking Time: 2 hours 35 minutes

Yields: 5 servings

Nutrition Facts: Calories: 868.8 | Carbs: 75.8g | Protein: 50.2g | Fat: 41.5g | Fiber: 14g

Ingredients:

- One big cabbage head (cut it into small wedges)
- Five peeled carrots (chopped into three-inch pieces)
- Ten red potatoes (small)
- Three pounds of corned beef brisket (along with the packet of spice)

Method:

1. At first, in a Dutch oven or a large pot, place the corned beef, and cover it with water. Then add in the spices from the packet of spices that came along with the beef. Cover the pot, bring it to a boil, and finally reduce it to a simmer. Allow it to simmer for about 2 hours and 30 minutes or until tender.

2. Add carrots and whole potatoes, and cook them until the vegetables are tender. Add the cabbage wedges and cook for another fifteen minutes. Then finally remove the meat and allow it to rest for fifteen minutes.

3. Take a bowl, place the vegetables in it, and cover it. Add broth (which is reserved in the pot) as much as you want. Then finally cut the meat against the grain.

Roasted Parsnips and Carrots

Total Prep & Cooking Time: 1 hour

Yields: 4 servings

Nutrition Facts: Calories: 112 | Carbs: 27g | Protein: 2g | Fat: 1g | Fiber: 7g

Ingredients:

- Two tbsps. of freshly minced parsley or dill
- One and a half tsp. of freshly ground black pepper
- One tbsp. kosher salt
- Three tbsps. of olive oil
- One pound of unpeeled carrots
- Two pounds of peeled parsnips

Method:

1. At first, preheat your oven to 425 degrees.

2. If the carrots and parsnips are thick, then cut them into halves lengthwise.

3. Then, slice each of them diagonally into one inch thick slices. Don't cut them too small because the vegetables will anyway shrink while you cook them.

4. Take a sheet pan, and place the cut vegetables on it.

5. Then add some olive oil, pepper, salt, and toss them nicely.

6. Roast them for about twenty to forty minutes (the roasting time depends on the size of the vegetables), accompanied by occasional tossing. Continue to roast until the carrots and parsnips become tender.

7. Finally, sprinkle some dill and serve.

Herbed Salmon

Total Prep & Cooking Time: 30 minutes

Yields: 4 servings

Nutrition Facts: Calories: 301 | Carbs: 1g | Protein: 29g | Fat: 19g | Fiber: 0g

Ingredients:

- Half a tsp. of dried thyme or two tsps. of freshly minced thyme
- Half a tsp. of pepper

- Three-fourth tsp. of salt
- One tbsp. of olive oil
- One tbsp. freshly minced rosemary or one tsp. of crushed dried rosemary.
- Four minced cloves of garlic
- Four (six ounces) fillets of salmon

Method:

1. At first, preheat your oven to 425 degrees.

2. Take a 15 by 10 by 1 inch baking pan and grease it.

3. Place the salmon on it while keeping the skin side down.

4. Combine the garlic cloves, rosemary, thyme, salt, and pepper. Spread it evenly over the salmon fillets.

5. Roast them for about fifteen to eighteen minutes until they reach your desired doneness.

Chipotle Cauliflower Tacos

Total Prep & Cooking Time: 30 minutes

Yields: 8 servings

Nutrition Facts: Calories: 440 | Carbs: 51.6g | Protein: 10.1g | Fat: 24g | Fiber: 9g

Ingredients:

For the tacos,

- Four tablespoons of avocado oil
- One head of cauliflower (large-sized, chopped into bite-sized florets)
- One cup of cilantro (freshly chopped)
- One tablespoon each of
  o Fresh lime juice
  o Maple syrup or honey
- Two tsps. of chipotle adobo sauce
- Cracked black pepper
- One teaspoon of salt
- 4-8 units of garlic cloves (freshly minced)

For the Chipotle Aioli,

- A quarter cup of chipotle adobo sauce
- Half a cup each of
  o Sour cream
  o Clean mayo
One teaspoon of sea salt

Two cloves of garlic (minced)

For serving,

- Almond flour tortillas
- Guacamole
- Almond ricotta cheese
- Sliced tomatoes, radish, and cabbage

Method:

1. Set the temperature of the oven to 425 degrees F. Now, use parchment paper to line a pan. Take the bite-sized florets of the cauliflower and spread them evenly on the pan. Use 2-4 tbsps. of avocado oil, pepper, salt, and minced garlic and drizzle it on the pan.

2. Roast the cauliflower for half an hour at 425 degrees F and halfway through the process, flip the florets.

3. When you are roasting the cauliflower, take the rest of the ingredients of the cauliflower and mix them in a bowl. Once everything has been properly incorporated, set the mixture aside.

4. Now, take another bowl and in it, add the ingredients of the chipotle aioli. Mix them and set the bowl aside.

5. If you have any other taco fixings, get them ready.

6. Once the cauliflower is ready, toss the florets in the chipotle sauce.

7. Serve the cauliflower in tortillas along with fixings of your choice and the chipotle aioli.

PART II

Be gentle with yourself throughout this process as it will be uncomfortable at times and will require strength. This book will help you through it, as you are not alone. I hope that this book also reminds you that many other people are suffering from the same type of food-related disorders as you are and that you are not alone in that either. This book will take a step-by-step approach, which will make for the highest chance of recovery. If at any time you need to take a break in order to think about the information you have learned, feel free to do so, but make sure you come back to this book quite soon after. Going through this process of recovery can be a lot, but with the right support, it will be possible.

You have already taken the first step in recovery, which is acknowledging that you have an issue. For that, I congratulate you!

What Is Emotional Eating?

Emotional eating occurs when a person suffering from emotional deficiencies of some sort, including lack of affection, lack of connection, or other factors like stress, depression, anxiety, or even general negative feelings like sadness or anger, eats in order to gain comfort from the food they are eating.

Many people find comfort in food. When people experience negative feelings and turn to food consumption in order to reduce their pain or to feel better, this is called emotional eating.

Now, some people do this on occasion like after a breakup or after a bad fight, but when this occurs at least a few times a week, this is when it is considered to have a negative impact on one's life and is when it becomes an issue that needs to be addressed.

What Is Binge Eating?

Binge eating disorder is another disorder that can be seen along with emotional eating. Binge eating disorder is when a person eats much more than a regular amount of food in a single occasion or sitting, and they feel unable to control themselves or to stop themselves. This could also be defined as a compulsion to overeat. In order to be considered a disorder, it has to happen at least two times per week for longer than six months consecutively.

Along with binge eating is overeating, although this is also sometimes seen as a separate disorder altogether. Overeating is when a person eats more than they require in order to sustain life. This occurs when they consume much more than they need in a day, or in a single sitting.

Overeating does not necessarily become binge eating, but it certainly can. Overeating is a general term used to describe the eating disorders that we just defined-Emotional Eating and Binge Eating. Thus, overeating could involve binge eating, food addiction, or other food-related disorders.

In this book, we will be focusing on emotional eating and binge eating, and how you can overcome these two food-related disorders.

What Is Bulimia?

Bulimia is another eating disorder. Bulimia involves binge eating, followed by extreme feelings of shame, guilt, and disdain for oneself and one's body. This is accompanied by intense feelings of body dysmorphia and body image issues, as well as the desire to be "skinnier." Thus, the person will turn to purging- or self-inflicted vomiting in an effort to lose weight and rid themselves of the guilt and shame.

Chapter 1: Understanding Your Food-Related Disorder

In this chapter, we are going to look at these two food-related disorders (binge eating/ bulimia and emotional eating) in much more detail. We will begin by looking at the most common reasons why people suffer from these disorders and will spend some time examining scientific research about why these disorders exist.

Why Do People Eat Emotionally?

The reason that emotional eating occurs is that eating foods that we enjoy makes us feel rewarded on an emotional and physiological level within our brain.

Why Do People Binge Eat?

People binge eat for a very similar reason to the reason why people experience emotional eating. This is because eating foods that we enjoy in terms of taste, smell, texture, and so on, makes us feel rewarded on an emotional and physiological level within our brains.

Throughout the rest of this chapter, we will look more in-depth at these eating disorders in order to give you more information about why they occur and what could cause them.

Scientific Research on Eating Disorders and Why They Exist

You may be asking how food cravings can result from emotional deficiencies and how these two seemingly unrelated things can be considered related. While we have touched on this briefly in this book already, the reason for this is that your body learns, over time, that eating certain foods makes it feel rewarding, positive, and happy for some time after it is ingested. These foods include convenience foods such as those containing processed sugars or salts, fast food, and quick pastries.

When you are sad or worried, your body feels negative and looks for ways to remedy this. Your brain then connects these two facts- that the body does not feel positive and that it wants to find a way to fix this. The brain then decides that eating the foods that make it feel good will remedy the situation. This process happens in the background of your mind without you being aware of it, and it leads you to consciously feel a craving for those specific foods such as sugary snacks or salty fast-food meals. You may not even be aware of why. If you then decide to give in to this craving and eat something like a microwave pizza snack, your body will feel rewarded and happy for a brief period of time. This reinforces to your brain that turning to food in an effort to make yourself feel better emotionally has been successful.

If you end up feeling down and guilty that you ate something that was unhealthy or that you ate too much, your brain will again try and remedy these negative emotions by craving food. This is how a cycle of emotional eating or a cycle of bingeing and purging can begin and continue. This could happen largely in your subconscious without you being any the wiser.

Why Do People Have Bulimia or Other Food Disorders?

Because scientists and psychiatrists understand this process that occurs in the brain, they know that food cravings can indicate emotional deficiencies. While there are other types of cravings that can occur, such as those that pregnant ladies experience, or those that indicate nutrient deficiencies, there are ways to tell that a craving is caused by some type of emotional deficiency.

It begins by determining the foods that a person craves and when they crave them. If every time someone has a stressful situation, they feel like eating a pizza, or if a person who is depressed tends to eat a lot of chocolate, this could indicate emotional eating. As you know by now, emotional eating and bulimia are closely related, and emotional eating can lead to bulimia over time.

If you crave fruit like a watermelon on a hot day, you are likely just dehydrated, and your body is trying to get water from a water-filled fruit that it knows will make it more hydrated. Examining situations like this has led scientists and psychiatrists to explore eating disorders in more depth and determine what types of emotional deficiencies can manifest themselves through food cravings or disordered eating in this way.

In the next chapter, we will look at psychological triggers that can lead to disordered eating.

The Neuroscience of Brain Chemicals and Food As a Reward

Many times, we may see ingredients on the packages of foods we eat, but we aren't really sure of exactly what they are, just that they taste good. In this section, we will take a deeper look at them and what they do to your brain.

Casein is a heavily processed ingredient that is derived from milk. It is processed a few times over and eventually creates milk solids that are concentrated. These milk solids- called Casein are then added into foods like cheese, french fries, milkshakes, and other fast and convenient packaged or fast-foods that contain dairy or dairy products (such as pastries and salad dressings). Casein has been compared to nicotine in its addictive properties. It is often seen in cheese, and this is why there is increasing evidence that people can become, and many are already addicted to cheese. The reason for this is during digestion. When cheese and other foods that contain casein are digested, it is broken down, and one of the compounds that it breaks down into is a compound that is strikingly similar to opioids- the highly addictive substance that is in pain killers.

High fructose corn syrup is surely an ingredient you have heard of before or at least one that you have seen on the packaging of your favorite snacks or quick foods. While this is actually derived from real corn, after it is finished being processed, there is nothing corn-like about it. High fructose corn syrup is essentially the same thing as refined sugar when all is said and done. It is used as a sweetener in foods like soda, cereal, and other sweet and quick foods. The reason why this ingredient is seen so often is that it is much cheaper than using sugar and is much easier to work with. High Fructose Corn Syrup is another common food additive that has been shown to be highly addictive. This substance has been shown to be similar to cocaine in its addictive properties.

MSG stands for Monosodium Glutamate, which sounds a lot like a chemical you may have encountered in science class in college. MSG is added to foods to give it a delicious flavor. It is essentially a very concentrated form of salt. What this does in foods such as fast-food, packaged convenience foods, and buffet-style food is that it gives it that wonderfully salty and fatty flavor that makes us keep coming back for more. Companies put this in food because it comes at an extremely low cost, and the flavor it brings covers up the artificial flavors of all of the other cheap ingredients that are used to make these foods. MSG has been known to block our natural appetite suppressant, which normally kicks in when we have had enough to eat. For this reason, when we are eating foods containing MSG, we do not recognize when we are satiated, and we continue to eat until we are stuffed because it tastes so great.

Chapter 2: Understanding Your Mind

In this chapter, we are going to look at some of the psychological factors that can lead to disordered eating so that you can gain a better understanding of what could have led you to use food as a means of coping.

Psychological and Emotional Triggers

There are several types of emotional deficiencies that can be indicated by disordered eating. We will explore these in detail below in hopes that you will recognize some of the reasons why you may be struggling with an eating disorder.

Childhood Causes

The first example of an emotional deficiency that we will examine is more of an umbrella for various emotional deficiencies. This umbrella term is Childhood Causes. If you think back on your childhood, think about how your relationship with food was cultivated. Maybe you were taught that when you behaved, you received food as a reward. Maybe when you were feeling down, you were given food to cheer you up. Maybe you turned to food when you were experiencing negative things in your childhood. Any of these could cause someone to suffer from emotional eating in their adulthood, as it had become something learned. This type is quite difficult to break as it has likely been a habit for many, many years, but it is possible. When we are children, we learn habits and make associations without knowing it that we often carry into our later lives. While this is no fault of yours, recognizing it as a potential issue is important to make changes.

Covering Up Emotions

Another emotional deficiency that can manifest itself in emotional eating and food cravings is actually the effort to cover up our emotions. Sometimes we would rather distract ourselves and cover up our emotions than to feel them or to face them head-on. In this case, our brain may make us feel hungry in an effort to distract us from the act of eating food. When we have a quiet minute where these feelings or thoughts would pop into our minds, we can cover them up by deciding to prepare food and eat and convince ourselves that we are "too busy" to acknowledge our feelings because we have to deal with our hunger. The fact that it is hunger that arises in this scenario makes it very difficult to ignore and very easy to deem as a necessary distraction since, after all, we do need to eat in order to survive. This can be a problem though, if we are not in need of nourishment, and we are telling ourselves that this is the reason why we cannot deal with our demons or our emotions. If there is something that you think you may be avoiding dealing with or thinking about or if you tend to be very uncomfortable with feelings of unrest, you may be experiencing this type of emotional eating.

Feeling Empty or Bored

When we feel bored, we often decide to eat or decide that we are hungry. This occupies our mind and our time and makes us feel less bored and even feel positive and happy. We also may eat when we are feeling empty. When we feel empty the food will quite literally be ingested in an effort to fill a void, but as we know, the food will not fill a void that is emotional in sort, and this will lead to an unhealthy cycle of trying to fill ourselves emotionally with something that will never actually work. This will lead us to become disappointed every time and continue trying to fill this void with material things like food or purchases. This can also be a general feeling of dissatisfaction with life and feelings of lacking something in your life. Looking deeper into this the next time you feel those cravings will be difficult but will help you greatly in the long term as you will then be able to identify the source of your feelings of emptiness and begin to fill these voids in ways that will be much more effective.

Affection Deficiency

Another emotional deficiency that could manifest itself as food cravings is an affection deficiency. This type of deficiency can be feelings of loneliness, feelings of a lack of love, or feelings of being undesired. If a person has been without an intimate relationship or has recently gone through a breakup, or if a person has not experienced physical intimacy in quite some time, they may be experiencing an affection deficiency. This type of emotional deficiency will often manifest itself in food cravings as we will try to gain feelings of comfort and positivity from the good tasting, drug-like (as we talked about in chapter one) foods they crave.

Low Self-Esteem

Another emotional deficiency that may be indicated by food cravings is a low level of self-esteem. Low self-esteem can cause people to feel down, unlovable, inadequate, and overall negative and sad. This can make a person feel like eating foods they enjoy will make them feel better, even if only for a few moments. Low self-esteem is an emotional deficiency that is difficult to deal with as it affects every area of a person's life, such as their love life, their social life, their career life, and so on. Sometimes people have reported feeling like food was something that was always there for them, and that never left them. While this is true, they will often be left feeling even emptier and lower about themselves after giving into cravings.

Mood

A general low mood can cause emotional eating. While the problem of emotional eating is something that is occurring multiple times per week and we all have general low moods or bad days, if this makes you crave food and especially food of an unhealthy sort, this could become emotional eating. If every time we feel down or are having a bad day, we want to eat food to make ourselves feel better; this is emotional eating. Some people will have a bad day and want a drink at the end of the day, and if this happens every once in a while, it is not necessarily a problem with emotional eating. The more often it happens, the more often it is emotional eating. Further, we do not have to give in to the cravings for it to be considered emotional eating. Experiencing the cravings often and in tandem with negative feelings in the first place is what constitutes emotional eating.

Depression

Suffering from depression also can lead to emotional eating. Depression is a constant low mood for a period of months on end, and this low mood can cause a person to turn to food for comfort and a lift in spirit. This can then become emotional eating in addition to and because of depression.

Anxiety

Having anxiety can lead to emotional eating, as well. There are several types of anxiety, and whether it is general anxiety (constant levels of anxiety), situational anxiety (triggered by a situation or scenario), it can lead to emotional eating. You have likely heard of the term *comfort food* to describe certain foods and dishes. The reason for this is because they are usually foods rich in carbohydrates, fats, and heavy in nature. These foods bring people a sense of comfort. These foods are often turned to when people suffering from anxiety are emotionally eating because these foods help to temporarily ease their anxiety and make them feel calmer and more at ease. This only lasts for a short period of time; however, before their anxiety usually gears up again.

Stress

Stress eating is probably the most common form of emotional eating. While this does not become an issue for everyone experiencing stress, and many people will do so every once in a while, it is a problem for those who consistently turn to food to ease their stress. Some people are always under stress, and they will constantly be looking for ways to ease their stress. Food is one of these ways that people use to make themselves feel better and to take their minds off of their stress. As with all of the other examples we have seen above, this is not a lasting resolution, and it becomes a cycle. Similar to the cycle diagram we saw above, the same can be used for stress except instead of a negative emotion and eating making you feel more down, stress eating can make you feel more stress as you feel like you have done something you shouldn't have which causes you stress, and the cycle ensues.

Recognizing your triggers is important because this will allow you to notice when you may be feeling emotional hunger and when you are feeling actual hunger. If you become hungry, you can look back on your day or on the last hour and determine if any of your triggers were present. If they were, then you will be able to determine that you are likely experiencing emotional hunger, and you can take the appropriate steps instead of giving in to the cravings blindly.

There are many different emotional causes for the cravings we experience. There may be others than those listed above, and these are all valid. A person's emotional eating experience is unique and personal and could be caused by any number of things. You may also experience a combination of emotional deficiencies listed above, or one of those listed above in addition to others. Many of these can overlap, such as anxiety and depression, which are often seen together in a single person. The level of these emotional deficiencies that you experience could indicate the level of emotional eating that you struggle with. Whatever your experience and your struggles though, there is hope of recovery, and this is what the rest of this book will focus on.

Chapter 3: How to Stop Binge Eating, Bulimia, and Emotional Eating

In this chapter, we are going to look at how you can begin to tackle your mind in order to make positive changes for your body and break free from your eating disorder once and for all.

Addressing the Core Wounds

The key to solving these food-related issues is to address your core wounds. Understanding how your mind works will help you to better take care of it. You will be able to recognize your feelings and how they could have come about, and then treat them in a way that will help it to feel better. Bettering your relationship with food and your body will also improve your relationship with your mind. This will then allow you to begin to feed it what it needs, which will, in turn, lead to better cognitive functioning, control over impulses, and decision-making. This will help overall in your relationship with your food, your body, and your mind.

What Are Core Wounds?

As we discussed in the previous chapter, there are several types of emotional deficiencies that can be indicated by disordered eating. Once you have determined which of these emotional deficiencies (or which combination of them) are present in your life, you can begin to look at them in a little more detail. By doing so, you will come upon your core wounds. A core wound is something that you believe to be true about yourself or your life, and it is something that likely came about as a result of a coping mechanism you developed to deal with childhood. For example, this could be something like; the feeling of not being enough, the belief that you are unlovable, or the belief that you are stupid.

How to Address Them

By understanding and addressing your core wounds, you will be able to change your behaviors because of the intricate relationship that exists between your thoughts, your emotions, and your behaviors. By addressing your thoughts and emotions, you will change your behaviors and thus, free yourself from disordered eating. You may be wondering how you can begin to address your core wounds, as it can be difficult to know where to begin.

The first step is learning how to control and change your thoughts, which in turn, leads to changes in your behavior. By taking control of your thoughts and your beliefs, they don't have the opportunity to manifest into unhealthy behaviors such as overeating, turning to food for comfort, or any other unhealthy coping mechanisms that you have developed over the course of your life.

Becoming aware of your own thoughts is the most crucial step in this entire guide, as everything else will fail without it. Paying attention to your thoughts will help you identify what thoughts are going through your mind during an intense emotional moment. By looking deep within, in order to get in touch with your deepest feelings, you will be more likely to succeed in your weight loss and your overall lifestyle improvement.

One great example of how to put this into practice is through the use of journaling. Journaling can help in a process such as this because it can help you to organize your thoughts and feelings and will help you to see visually what is working and what isn't working for you. While we can give tips and examples, every person is different, so to find exactly what works for you, you will have to try some different things and see which techniques help you personally the most and in the best way. Journaling can be about anything like how you feel since beginning a new program, how you feel physically since changing your diet, how you feel emotionally now that you are not reaching for food in order to comfort your emotions and anything along the lines of this.

Positive Self-Talk

Once you have addressed your emotions and your core wounds, you can begin to intervene and change them so that they result in healthier behaviors. You will do this using positive self-talk. Adopting helpful thought processes fosters better emotions overall, which leads to more productive behaviors.

When people have developed unhelpful thinking processes, it is hard to make decisions to benefit their future selves because their thoughts create negative emotions that drive away motivation. This is where something called *positive self-talk* can come in. Positive self-talk can be instrumental in helping you to recover from disordered eating.

What Is Positive Self-Talk?

Many people's minds are controlled by their inner critic. The inner critic shares words with you, such as "You should just give up" Or "What makes you think you'll succeed?" which is rooted in the opposite of positive self-talk- Negative self-talk!

Instead of creating an open space that allows for mistakes, growth, and development, your inner critic causes you to question your worth, which makes it difficult for you to have the positive, growth mindset that is needed to complete tasks and go after things that may be difficult to achieve. In this case, helping your mind to begin using positive self-talk will help you to recover for the long-term.

How to Use Positive Self-Talk?

Below are several ways that you can begin to use positive self-talk. Over time, your mind will get used to thinking in this way, and you will find it much easier to do.

1. Remind yourself

Bad habits are built through many years, and no amount of willpower can undo a lifetime of bad habits, such as a strong inner critic that uses negative self-talk. By rewiring your brain to minimize the amount of negativity you feel in the first place, you will eventually get used to filling your mind with positive thoughts instead of negative ones.

2. Stop the automatic process of negativity

Often times, if the person had just paid attention to their thought process, they would be able to catch themselves before their mind automatically spiraled to a place of complete de-motivation. By catching yourself before you get there, you can prevent yourself from falling into your negative thought patterns that are limiting you and holding you back.

3. Find positive influences

Surrounding yourself with people that can encourage you and foster positivity will also change your inner-critic's opinion. Often times, hearing positive compliments from other people hold a heavier weight in the eyes of your inner-critic compared to you telling your inner-critic the same thing. Try spending time with people who are supportive of your goals and the changes that you are looking to make in your life. It will make your journey a little bit easier.

4. Limit Negative Influences

By limiting the negative influences in your life, you are making a statement to yourself that you place importance on preserving your mental health. When you remove negative influences and limit your exposure to things or people that make you feel negative, you are prioritizing yourself, and this is a great way to practice self-care.

5. Practice a gratitude exercise

This is a great exercise to remind yourself of everything that you love and appreciate about yourself and your life. Take time to write down all of the things that you love about yourself and about your life. This will remind you of all of the positivity surrounding you and will serve to uplift you.

Chapter 4: Making Healthier Decisions Using Intuitive

Eating

This chapter will provide you with a solid foundation of knowledge on which to build your new lifestyle. We will look at how intuitive eating can be the answer to all of your struggles and help you to find recovery.

Making Good Choices

As we discussed in the previous chapter, making good choices begins with self-exploration and a deep look into your core wounds. Once you have done this, you can begin to make decisions that are positive for your health and your life, and over time these will become more and more habitual. We are going to spend this chapter looking at some of the ways that you can begin to make good choices related to food and eating.

How to Begin Making Good Choices Using Intuitive Eating

One great way to make good choices when it comes to food is by using something called intuitive eating. Below, I will define intuitive eating for you and give you some insight into how this can change your life.

What Is Intuitive Eating?

Intuitive eating is a new perspective from which to view how you feed your body. This style of eating puts you in control, instead of following a list of pre-designed guidelines about when and what to eat. Intuitive eating instead encourages you to listen to your body and the signals it sends you about what, how much, and when to eat. This ensures that you are giving your body exactly what it needs when it needs it, instead of forcing it into a specific kind of diet.

Intuitive eating does not limit any specific foods and does not require you to stick to certain foods exclusively. Instead, it encourages you to learn as much as you can about what your body is telling you and follow its signals.

The two main components of the intuitive eating philosophy are the following; eat when you are hungry and stop eating when you are satiated. This may seem like a no-brainer, but in today's societies, we are very far from eating in an intuitive way, as odd as it may seem. With so many diet trends and numerous "rules" for how you should and should not eat, it can be difficult to put these ideas aside and let your body guide you exclusively.

Intuitive Eating and Hunger

Before we begin looking at the specifics of intuitive eating, we will look at the different types of hunger and how you can tell them apart. This will help you to distinguish when you are hungry and when you may be turning to food to soothe your emotional state.

Real hunger is when our body needs nutrients or energy and is letting us know that we should replenish our energy soon. This happens when it has been a few hours since our last meal when we wake up in the morning, or after a lot of strenuous activity like a long hike. Our body uses hunger to signal to us that it is in need of more energy and that if it doesn't get it soon, it will begin to use our stored energy as fuel. While there is nothing wrong with our body using its stored fuel, it can be used as a sign to us that we should eat shortly in order to replenish these stores. Perceived Hunger is when we think we are hungry, but our body doesn't actually require any more energy or for the stores to be replenished. This can happen for a number of reasons, including an emotional deficiency, a negative mental state, or the occurrence of a psychological trigger.

The philosophy behind intuitive eating is that if you wait until you are too hungry before eating, you will be much more likely to overeat or to binge eat. This is because, by this time, you be feeling ravenous instead of mildly hungry. If instead, you choose to adhere to your hunger and eat when your body tells you that it needs sustenance, you will be much more likely to eat just the right amount. As a result, your body will be satisfied rather than completely stuffed, and instead of feeling shameful and angry that you have eaten, you can feel happy that you have provided your body with what it needed. This requires you to listen to and respect what your body is telling you and then provide it with nutrients in order for it to keep working hard for you!

The Benefits of Intuitive Eating

One of the reasons that intuitive eating is such a successful and cherished form of eating is that it allows the body to lead the mind in the right direction when it comes to seeking out its needs. Below, we will look at the benefits of letting your body guide your eating choices.

- Allows the body to get what it needs

Did you know that your cravings could actually be giving you much more information than you give them credit for?

A craving is an intense longing for something (in this case food), that comes about intensely and feels urgent. In our case, that longing is for s a very specific type of food. When we have cravings for certain foods, it can actually mean more than what it seems.

While you may think that a craving is an indication of hunger or of a desire for the taste of a certain food, it may actually indicate that your body is low on certain vitamins or minerals. As a result, your body seeks out a certain food that it thinks will provide it with this vitamin or mineral. This reaches your consciousness in the form of an intense craving. In this case, the body is trying to help itself by telling you what to eat. For this reason, understanding your cravings could help you give your body exactly what it is longing for.

For example, if you are craving juice or pop or other sugary drinks like this, consider that you might actually be dehydrated and, therefore, thirsty. Sometimes we see drinks in our fridge, and since we are thirsty, we really want them. Next time you are craving a sugary drink, try having a glass of water first, then wait a few minutes and see if you are still craving that Coca-Cola. You may not want it anymore once your thirst is quenched.

If you are craving meat, you may feel like you want some fried chicken or a hot dog. This can indicate a deficit of iron or protein. The best sources of protein are chicken breast cooked in the oven, and iron is best received from spinach, oysters, or lentils. If you think you may not like these foods, there are many different ways to prepare them, and you can likely find a way that you like.

- Prevents overeating

It can be hard to know how much to eat and when you have had enough to eat without letting yourself eat too much. Sometimes people will eat until the point that they begin to feel completely full. Many times, we keep eating until we become stuffed, even to the point of making ourselves feel physically ill. Intuitive eating will help you to avoid this, as this kind of eating encourages you to give your body what it needs in order to take great care of it. Stuffing your body until it is too full is not what your body is asking for, and once you become accustomed to listening to your body's needs, you will know when it is time to stop.

- Helps you break free from self-judgment

intuitive eating will help you to finally make peace with your body and yourself as a whole. It does this by showing you that your body has needs and that there is no shame in tending to these needs, as long as you do so in a healthy way.

You cannot fully embrace and practice intuitive eating if you have those nagging feelings of self-judgment each time you take a bite of food or decide that you are going to eat lunch when you are hungry. For this reason, in order to practice intuitive eating, you must understand that feeding your body is an act of compassion for yourself and that this does not need to come with self-judgment.

- It is inclusive, not exclusive

One of the great things about this style of eating is that it is not founded on restricting a person's intake of certain foods or allowing only a small variety of foods.

Diets like this are extremely hard to transition to and are hard to maintain for a long period of time. Intuitive eating is about including as many natural whole foods as you wish, while also ensuring that you are consuming enough of all of your nutrients. With this style of eating, you can eat whatever you wish, whenever you wish. This makes it much easier to stick with this type of diet and reduces the chances of falling off after a short period of time due to cravings or intense hunger. It does not restrict calories or reduce your intake greatly, which makes it easier to handle than a traditional diet for many people. It feels natural to eat in this way, which makes it effective.

Chapter 5: Intuitive Eating Part 2

In this chapter, we are going to continue our examination of intuitive eating by looking at some more specific details related to this diet, as well as how to make it a regular part of your life.

How to Make Intuitive Eating Part of Your Life

One of the best ways to make this type of eating a part of your life is to practice it with intention. This is especially important when you are just beginning. Each time you feel a pang of hunger or a compulsion to eat, take a minute to examine your inner world. By doing this, you will get your mind and body accustomed to working together. In addition, do the same after you eat. By doing these two things, you will be able to ensure that you are eating when hungry and stopping when satisfied.

When you finish eating a meal, rank your level of fullness on a scale of 1 to 10, 1 being extremely hungry and 10 being extremely stuffed. This will help you to determine if you are successfully stopping when you are satisfied and not overeating.

It is also important that you learn how to deal with your emotions and feelings in an effective way without using food. Using the techniques that you have learned in this book, you will be able to address your inner demons, which will make space for you to listen to your body and its needs.

As you know by now, listening to your body, your emotions and your mind is extremely important when it comes to practicing intuitive eating. As long as you remember this, you will be well on your way to becoming a lifelong intuitive eater.

What Kind of Foods Should You Choose?

Fish is a great way to get healthy fats into your diet. Certain fish are very low in carbohydrates but high in good fats, making them perfect for a healthy diet. They also contain minerals and vitamins that will be good for your health. Salmon is a great fish to eat, as it is versatile and delicious. Many fish also include essential fatty acids that we can only get through our diet. Other fish that are good for you include:

- Sardines
- Mackerel
- Herring
- Trout
- Albacore Tuna

Meat and Poultry make up a large part of most Americans' diets. Meats and poultry that are fresh and not processed do not include any carbohydrates and contain high levels of protein. Eating lean meats helps to maintain your strength and muscle mass and gives you energy for hours. Grass-fed meats, in particular, are rich in antioxidants.

Eggs are another amazing, protein-filled food. Eggs help your body to feel satiated for longer and also keeps your blood sugar levels consistent, which is great for overall health. The whole egg is good for you, as the yolk is where the nutrients are. The cholesterol found within egg yolks also has been demonstrated to lower your risk of getting diseases like heart diseases, despite what most people think. Therefore, do not be afraid of the egg yolk!

Legumes are a great source of protein as well as fiber, and there are many different types to choose from. These include the following:

- All sorts of beans including black beans, green beans, and kidney beans
- Peas
- Lentils of all colors
- Chickpeas
- Peas

Examples of fruits that you can eat include the following:

- Citrus fruits such as oranges, grapefruits, lemons, and limes
- Melons of a variety of sorts
- Apples
- Bananas
- Berries including strawberries, blueberries, blackberries, raspberries and so on
- Grapes

Vegetables are a great source of energy and nutrients, and they include a wide range of naturally occurring vivid colors which should all be included in your diet.

- Carrots
- Broccoli and cauliflower
- Asparagus
- Kale
- All sorts of peppers including hot peppers, bell peppers
- Tomatoes

- Root vegetables (that are a good source of healthy, complete carbohydrates) such as potatoes, sweet potatoes, all types of squash, and beets.

Seeds are another great source of nutrients, vitamins, and minerals, and they are very versatile. These include the following:

- Sesame seeds
- Pumpkin seeds
- Sunflower seeds
- Hemp, flax and chia seeds are all especially good for your health

Nuts are a great way to get protein if you are choosing not to eat meat or if you are vegan. They also are packed with nutrients. Some examples are below.

- Almonds
- Brazil Nuts
- Cashews
- Macadamia nuts
- Pistachios
- Pecans

There are some **healthy fats** that are essential components of any person's diet, as the beneficial compounds that they contain cannot be made by our bodies; thus, we rely solely on or diet to get them. These compounds are Omega-3 Fatty Acids, monounsaturated and polyunsaturated fats. Below are some healthy sources of these compounds:

- Avocados

- Healthy, plant-based oils including olive oil and canola oil
- Hemp, chia and flax seeds
- Walnuts

When it comes to carbohydrates, these should be consumed in the form of **whole grains**, as they are high in fiber, which will help to prevent overeating. Whole grains also include essential minerals- those that we can only get from our diet just like those essential compounds found in healthy fats. These essential minerals are selenium, magnesium, and copper. Sources of these whole grains include the following:

- Quinoa
- Rye, Barley, buckwheat
- Whole grain oats
- Brown rice
- Whole grain bread can be hard to find these days in the grocery store, as many brown breads disguise themselves as whole grain when, in fact, they are not. However, there are whole grain breads if you take the time to look at the ingredients list.

Nutrients You Need and How to Get Them

In this section, we are going to look at the most beneficial nutrients for your body and where/ how you can find them. This will help you to decide which foods to include in your diet so that you can ensure you are getting all of the nutrients that your body needs.

1. Omega-3 Fatty Acids

Some vitamins and nutrients are called "essential nutrients." Omega-3 Fatty Acids are an example of this type of nutrient. They are called essential nutrients because they cannot be made by our bodies; thus, they must be eaten in our diets. These fatty acids are a very specific type of fatty acid, and this type, in particular, is the most essential and the most beneficial for our brains and bodies.

They have numerous effects on the brain, including reducing inflammation (which reduces the risk of Alzheimer's) and maintaining and improving mood and cognitive function, including specifically memory. Omega-3's have these greatly beneficial effects because of the way that they act in the brain, which is what makes them so essential to our diets. Omega-3 Fatty Acids increase the production of new nerve cells in the brain by acting specifically on the nerve stem cells within the brain, causing new and healthy nerve cells to be generated.

Omega-3 fatty acids can be found in fish like salmon, sardines, black cod, and herring. It can also be taken as a pill-form supplement for those who do not eat fish or cannot eat enough of it. It can also be taken in the form of a fish oil supplement like krill oil.

Omega-3 is by far the most important nutrient that you need to ensure you are ingesting because of the numerous benefits that come from it, both in the brain and in the rest of the body. While supplements are often a last step when it comes to trying to include something in your diet, for Omega-3's, the benefits are too great to potentially miss by trying to receive all of it from your diet.

Magnesium

Magnesium is beneficial for your diet, as it also helps you to maintain strong bones and teeth. Magnesium and Calcium are most effective when ingested together, as Magnesium helps in the absorption of calcium. It also helps to reduce migraines and is great for calmness and relieving anxiety. Magnesium can be found in leafy green vegetables like kale and spinach, as well as fruits like bananas and raspberries, legumes like beans and chickpeas, vegetables like peas, cabbage, green beans, asparagus, and brussels sprouts, and fish like tuna and salmon.

Calcium

Calcium is beneficial for the healthy circulation of blood, and for maintaining strong bones and teeth. Calcium can come from dairy products like milk, yogurt, and cheese. It can also be found in leafy greens like kale and broccoli and sardines.

Chapter 6: How to Make These New Choices a Habit

Now that you have learned a wealth of information about intuitive eating, we are going to look at some strategies that you can use to make these new, healthy choices a habit. This will take time, but by employing these strategies, you will surely find success.

Healthy Thinking Patterns

In this section, we will look at a real-life example of dealing with challenges to demonstrate healthy thinking patters when it comes to intuitive eating.

Let's say you are trying to focus on healthy eating, and you find that you have had trouble doing so. Maybe you ate a cupcake, or maybe you had a soda at breakfast. From the perspective of traditional diet mentality, this would become a problem for the diet, and this would become a problem in your mind as well. You would likely be beating yourself up and feeling terrible about the choice you have made.

Let's look at this example in more detail. It is very important to avoid beating yourself up or self-judging for falling off the wagon. This may happen sometimes. What we need to do though, is to focus not on the fact that it has happened, but on how we are going to deal with and react to it. There are a variety of reactions that a person may have to this type of situation. We will examine the possible reactions and their pros and cons below:

- You may feel as though your progress is ruined and that you might as well begin again another time. This could lead you to go back to your old ways and keep you from trying again for quite some time. This could happen many times, over and over again, and each time you slip up, you decide that you might as well give up this time and try again, but each time it ends the same.

- You may fall off of your plan and tell yourself that this day is a write-off and that you will begin again the next day. The problem with this method is that continuing the rest of the day as you would have before you decided to make a change will make it so that the next day is like beginning all over again, and it will be very hard to begin again. You may be able to begin again the next day, and it could be fine, but you must be able to really motivate yourself if you are going to do this. Knowing that you have fallen off before makes it so that you may feel down on yourself and feel as though you can't do it, so beginning again the next day is very important.

- The third option, similar to the previous case, you may fall off, but instead of deciding that the day is a write-off, you tell yourself that the entire week is a write-off, and you then decide that you will pick it up again the next week. This will be even harder than starting again the next day as multiple days of eating whatever you like will make it very hard to go back to making the healthy choices again afterward.

- After eating something that you wish you hadn't (and that wasn't a healthy choice), you decide not to eat anything for the rest of the day so that you don't eat too many calories or too much sugar, and decide that the next day you will start over again. This is very difficult on the body as you are going to be quite hungry by the time the evening rolls around. Instead of forgiving yourself, you are punishing yourself, and it will make it very hard not to reach for chips late at night when you are starving and feeling down.

- The fifth and final option is what you should do in this situation.

This option is the best for success and will make it the most likely that you will succeed long-term. If you fall off at lunch, let's say, because you are tired and, in a rush, and you just grab something from a fast-food restaurant instead of going home for lunch or buying something at the grocery store to eat, this is how we will deal with it. Firstly, you will likely feel like you have failed and may feel quite down about having made an unhealthy choice. Now instead of starving for the rest of the day or eating only lettuce for dinner, you will put this slip up at lunch behind you, and you will continue your day as if it never happened. You will eat a healthy dinner as you planned, and you will continue on with the plan. You will not wait until tomorrow to begin again; you will continue as you would if you had made that healthy choice at lunch. The key to staying on track is being able to bounce back. The people who can bounce back mentally are the ones who will be most likely to succeed. You will need to maintain a positive mental state and look forward to the rest of the day and the rest of the week in just the same way as you did before you had a slip-up. One bad meal out of the entire week is not going to ruin all of your progress and recovering from emotional eating is largely a mental game. It is more mental than anything else, so we must not underestimate the role that our mindset plays in our success or failure.

By using this type of thinking, you will set yourself up for success and will not fall off of your plan completely after one slip up.

Healthy Lifestyle Changes

One important way to ensure that these healthy choices stick for good is by changing some aspects of your lifestyle. By doing this, you will reduce the chances of slipping up by eliminating them altogether. For example, you can change the way you approach the grocery store.

When you are entering the grocery store, it is important that you change a few things about the way you shop, in order to set yourself up for success. This is especially important when you are just beginning your intuitive eating practice, as it will be challenging for you to enter the grocery store and avoid cravings and temptations.

The first thing to keep in mind when grocery shopping for a new diet is to enter with a list. By doing this, you are giving yourself a guide to follow, which will prevent you from picking up things that you are craving or things that you feel like eating in that moment.

One of the biggest things to keep in mind when beginning a new eating practice like intuitive eating is to avoid shopping when you are hungry. This will make you reach for anything and everything that you see. By entering the grocery store when you are satiated or when you have just eaten, you will be able to stick to your list and avoid falling prey to temptations.

If you treat your grocery shopping experience like a treasure hunt, you will be able to cross things off of the list one at a time without venturing to the parts of the grocery store that will prove to be a challenge for you to resist. If you are making healthy eating choices, you will likely be spending most of your time at the perimeter of the grocery store. This is where the whole, plant-based foods are located. By doing this, and entering with a list, you will be able to avoid the middle aisles where the processed, high-sugar temptation foods are all kept.

Having a plan is key when it comes to succeeding in learning new habits and employing a new lifestyle. This plan can be as detailed as you wish, or it can simply come in the form of a general overview. I recommend you start with a more detailed plan in the beginning as you ease into things.

As everyone is different, you may be the type of person who likes lots of lists and plans, or you may be the type of person who doesn't, but for everyone, beginning with a plan and following it closely for the first little while is best. For example, this plan can include things like what you will focus on each week, what you will reduce your intake of, and what you will try to achieve in terms of the mental work involved.

Once you have come up with a general plan for your new lifestyle and how you want it to look, you can then begin laying out more specific plans.

Planning your individual meals will make it much easier for you when you get home from work or when you wake up tired in the morning and need to pack something for your lunch.

You can plan your meals out a week in advance, two weeks or even a month if you wish. You can post this up on your fridge, and each day you will know exactly what you are eating, with no thinking required. This way, there won't be a chance for you to consider ordering a pizza or heating up some chicken fingers because you will already know exactly what you are going to make. By approaching your new style of eating in this way, you can make this transition easier on yourself and ensure success every step of the way.

30-Day Meal Plan

The following 30-day meal plan includes a variety of meals that you can make in order to keep your first thirty days interesting and tasty!

Day 1

- Breakfast:

Coffee

Feta, mushroom and spinach, omelet.

- Lunch:

Oven-baked tempeh with broccoli and cauliflower rice.

- Dinner:

Chicken Caesar salad- tofu and romaine lettuce, parmesan

Day 2

- Breakfast:

Unsweetened yogurt with a mix of some berries such as strawberries, raspberries, and some seeds like flax seeds and chia seeds, and nuts like sliced almonds and walnuts.

- Lunch:

A healthy lunch-time salad with avocado, cheese, grape tomatoes, and a variety of nuts and seeds like spicy pumpkin seeds. Add a salad dressing on top such as blue cheese or ranch dressing, or a homemade one using olive oil and garlic.

- Dinner:

Chicken breast with onions and a homemade tomato sauce. Served alongside some grilled zucchini or eggplant.

Day 3

- Breakfast:

A no sugar added full fat Greek yogurt bowl with seeds, nuts and berries.

1 Cup of coffee

- Lunch:

Make your own lunch box, including firm tofu or meat of some sort, raw tomatoes, any type of cheese cubes that you wish, pickles, a hard-boiled egg, vegetables such as celery, carrots, radishes or zucchini, nuts for protein and fat such as walnuts, or almonds, homemade guacamole (avocado, onion, garlic, jalapeno).

- Dinner:

Grilled portobello, grilled eggplant and grilled zucchini as well as cherry tomatoes sautéed in extra virgin olive oil with garlic. Served with rice and protein such as pork or chicken.

Day 4

- Breakfast:

Coffee

Homemade mushroom & Spinach Frittata, including any vegetables that you wish such as bell peppers and onion.

- Lunch:

Cream cheese with cucumber slices for dipping.

Hard-boiled egg

Meatballs with sweet and sour sauce

- Dinner

Bacon, Avocado, Lettuce, Tomato panini.

Day 5

- Breakfast:

Egg Salad with lettuce, cucumber and whole grain bread.

- Lunch:

Homemade guacamole (avocado, onion, garlic, jalapeno, lime juice) with raw zucchini slices for dipping.

Hard-boiled egg

Tuna

- Dinner:

Cauliflower gratin (cheese, cauliflower, onion, garlic and so on)

As well as chopped lettuce drizzled with Caesar Dressing

Day 6

- Breakfast:

Coffee with heavy cream or coconut oil.

Celery sticks, dipped in peanut or Almond Butter

- Lunch:

Leftover cauliflower gratin

As well as chopped lettuce drizzled with Caesar Dressing

- Dinner:

Cooked or raw broccoli with grated cheese on top

Steak seared in olive oil

Day 7

- Breakfast:

Pancakes with fresh fruits

Black Coffee

- Lunch:

Cold pasta salad with fresh vegetables

Feta and Tomato Meatballs

Raw fresh spinach

- Dinner:

Spicy Spaghetti Squash Casserole

Fresh spinach, raw or cooked with 1 Tbsp ranch dressing drizzled on top.

Day 8

- Breakfast

Smoothie

- Lunch

Tempeh meatballs with guacamole and raw vegetable salad

- Dinner

Rice noodle stir fry with your choice of vegetables and tofu

Day 9

- Breakfast

Omelet cooked in coconut oil with cheese, onions, bell pepper and tomatoes

- Lunch

Tofu scramble with vegetables such as spinach and mushrooms and cheese

- Dinner

Curry with chicken, rice and coconut milk sauce with hot chili paste

Day 10

- Breakfast

Full fat yogurt unsweetened with berries, chia seeds, flax seeds

- Lunch

Cobb salad with boiled egg, vegetables of your choice, tofu, tempeh or chicken and Caesar dressing

- Dinner

Homemade pizza with your choice of toppings

Day 11

- Breakfast

Smoothie with chia seeds and flax seeds, berries and plant-based protein powder, as well as plant-based milk

- Lunch

Salad with tofu or boiled egg, olive oil dressing, spinach and diced vegetables

- Dinner

Vegetarian frittata using coconut oil, spinach, mushroom, cheese, bell peppers and tomato

Day 12

- Breakfast

Greek yogurt no sugar added with nuts and seeds

- Lunch

Homemade tacos with your choice of toppings, including ground turkey

- Dinner

Macaroni and cheese with crumbled roasted bread crumbs on top

Day 13

- Breakfast

Whole grain oats with no sugar added, nuts, flax and chia seeds as well as heavy cream and a plant-based nut butter.

- Lunch

Lettuce wraps with curried tofu and grilled eggplant and zucchini

- Dinner

Homemade burritos filled with crumbled, seasoned meat of your choice, sour cream, guacamole and diced tomatoes

Day 14

- Breakfast

Greek yogurt no sugar added with nuts and seeds

- Lunch

Avocado egg bowls with bacon

- Dinner

Fried rice with your choice of vegetables, scrambled egg and tofu

Day 15

- Breakfast

Coffee with heavy cream and no sugar added

- Lunch

Carrots with guacamole, cottage cheese with nuts and seeds and homemade baked zucchini chips with olive oil drizzle

- Dinner

Egg Salad with Lettuce Wraps

Day 16

- Breakfast

Pancakes with no sugar added maple syrup

- Lunch

Vegetarian egg quiche with spinach and mushroom

- Dinner

Broccoli salad with onion, a cheese of your choice, creamy ranch dressing, almonds and walnuts sliced, as well as some avocado and tofu cubes

Day 17

- Breakfast

Potato hash browns fried in olive oil, sunny side up egg and tempeh "bacon" with a side of grilled tomatoes

- Lunch

Avocadoes stuffed with cauliflower "taco meat", homemade salsa with tomatoes and herbs, sour cream, and grated cheese

- Dinner

Cooked or raw broccoli

Small amount of butter that can be added to the broccoli for taste

Grated cheese on top that can also be added to the broccoli

With steak seared in olive oil

Day 18

- Breakfast

Shakshuka with eggs, tomatoes and parsley

- Lunch

Grilled zucchini roll ups with tomato and cheese

- Dinner

Coconut milk curry with rice, bell peppers and tofu

Day 19

- Breakfast

Breakfast smoothie with berries, no sugar added and full fat milk

- Lunch

Broccoli and cheese fritters with homemade hummus to dip and a side of carrots, celery and cucumber for dipping

- Dinner

Cobb salad including hard-boiled egg, ham cubes, your choice of vegetables and an olive oil or ranch dressing

Day 20

- Breakfast

Spinach and mushroom frittata

- Lunch

Sandwich with scrambled eggs, spinach and mushrooms cooked in olive oil and topped with lettuce, tomato or any other fillings or toppings you wish to include. Finally, add a homemade creamy avocado sauce with avocado, cilantro, pepper and salt and some sour cream.

- Dinner

Rice risotto with cheese, vegetable broth and mushrooms

Day 21

- Breakfast

Unsweetened yogurt with a mix of berries such as strawberries, raspberries, and some seeds like flax seeds and chia seeds, and nuts like sliced almonds and walnuts.

- Lunch

Caesar salad- dressing with no sugar added

Raw vegetables, mixed greens and tempeh

- Dinner

Cauliflower gratin- cheese, cauliflower and choice of vegetables

Day 22

- Breakfast

Hash browns fried in olive oil, sunny side up egg and bacon with a side of grilled tomatoes

- Lunch

Stuffed half zucchini with feta cheese, tomato sauce (no sugar added) and herbs for topping

- Dinner

Mashed potatoes using whole milk and cheese, with grilled eggplant and mushrooms

Day 23

- Breakfast

Nut butter smoothie with yogurt, nut butter, flax seeds, chia seeds

- Lunch

Pan fried steak seasoned with herbs and olive oil, paired with

A spinach salad with raw vegetables of choice and no sugar added Caesar dressing

- Dinner

Cauliflower pasta salad with celery, spinach, onions, and walnuts

Day 24

- Breakfast

Feta, mushroom and Spinach, omelet

Coffee

- Lunch

Coleslaw with a creamy cilantro dressing, carrots, cabbage, celery, tomato and herbs for topping

- Dinner

Crispy tofu cubes with zucchini noodles and a homemade peanut sauce

Day 25

- Breakfast

No bake protein bars

Coffee with no sugar added

- Lunch

Roasted tomatoes with goat cheese, spinach, cilantro and olive oil & balsamic drizzle

- Dinner

Eggplant and zucchini "French fries" with olive oil and crispy tofu cubes

Baked chicken breast

Day 26

- Breakfast

Pancakes with no sugar added maple syrup, full fat Greek yogurt and berries for topping

- Lunch

Low carb broccoli cheese soup with crispy cauliflower on the side

- Dinner

Curried rice with choice of vegetables, such as bell peppers and broccoli

Day 27

- Breakfast

Breakfast salad with scrambled egg, avocado, mixed greens, grilled tomatoes and cheese

- Lunch

Fried goat cheese with roasted red peppers, spinach and olive oil drizzle

- Dinner

Spicy Spaghetti Squash Casserole

Fresh spinach, raw or cooked with ranch dressing drizzled on top

Day 28

- Breakfast

Full fat yogurt unsweetened with berries, chia seeds, flax seeds

- Lunch

Vegetarian chili with tomato, sour cream, a variety of beans and tomatoes

- Dinner

Zucchini spiral pasta noodles with creamy yogurt avocado sauce

Day 29

- Breakfast

Cauliflower "bread" grilled cheese sandwich (similar to cauliflower crust pizza but made as a grilled cheese sandwich instead.

- Lunch

Green beans with mushrooms and tomatoes with a chicken breast on the side

- Dinner

Grape tomato marinara on pasta noodles with parmigiano Reggiano cheese and fresh cracked pepper.

Day 30

- Breakfast

Egg taco shells filled with choice of vegetables

- Lunch

Baked crispy tofu steaks with a sesame seed crust on a bed of zucchini strips and spinach

- Dinner

Baked Spaghetti squash filled with roasted tomatoes and eggplant, topped with melted, crispy cheese

Chapter 7: What to Do Next

As you take all of this information forth with you, it may seem overwhelming to begin applying this to your own life. Remember, life is a process, and you do not need to expect perfection from yourself right away. By taking the first step-reading this book, you are already on your way to changing your life. If you fall off and find that you are back to your old ways, try to find inspiration in the pages of this book once again. If you find that you are unable to find success on your own, there is no shame in seeking professional help. There are many people who are trained professionals in dealing with disordered eating and who can serve as a mentor or a guide for you as you navigate this challenge.

How To Seek Help If It Becomes Uncontrollable?

Understanding and accepting that you need help is the first step to recovery. By reading this book, you have taken this step. If you need further help, there is no shame in accepting this fact. There are many ways to seek help for disordered eating, depending on the level of help that you need. Below is a list of ways that you can seek help, ordered from least to most help.

- Online resources
- Support System
- Support Group
- Group counseling
- Anonymous online counseling or telephone counseling
- One on One counseling

- Talk therapy
- Rehab centers

Counseling or Therapy

Talking therapies are very effective treatments for disordered eating. The things that people learn in therapy gives them the insight and skills in order to feel better and tackle their eating disorder, as well as to prevent it from coming back in the future.

One example of talk therapy is Cognitive Behavioral Therapy or CBT. The way that cognitive behavioral therapy works is by putting an emphasis on the relationship between a person's thoughts, emotions, and behaviors. The theory behind this is that when a person changes any one of these components, change will be initiated in the others. The goal of CBT is to help a person decrease negative thoughts or the amount of worry they experience in order to increase their overall quality of life.

If you think that this is something you would benefit from, please reach out to your local resources to find out more.

PART III

The sirtfood diet is one of the latest diet patterns that has garnered quite the attention. The idea was brought to the market by two nutritionists Glen Matten and Aidan Goggins. The main idea of the diet revolves around sirtuins, which are basically a group of 7 proteins that are responsible for the functioning and regulation of lifespan, inflammation, and metabolism (Sergiy Libert, 2013).

Chapter 1: Health Benefits of the Diet

The benefits are vast. This includes loss in weight, better skin quality, gain in muscle mass in the areas that are very much required, increased metabolic rate, feeling of fullness without having to eat much (this is the power of the foods actually), suppressing the appetite, and leading a better and confident life. This specifically includes an increase in the memory, supporting the body to control blood sugar and blood cholesterol level in a much-advanced way, and wiping out the damage caused by the free radicals and thus preventing them from having adverse impacts on the cells that might lead to other diseases like cancer.

The consumption of these foods, along with the drinks, has a number of observational shreds of evidence that link the sirtfoods with the reducing hazards of several chronic diseases. This diet is notably suited as an anti-aging scheme. Sirtfoods have the ability to satiate the appetite in a natural way and increase the functioning of the muscle. These two points are enough to find a solution that can ultimately help us to achieve a healthy weight. In addition to this, the health-improving impact of these compounds is powerful in comparison to the drugs that are prescribed in order to prevent several chronic diseases like that of diabetes, heart problems, Alzheimer's, etc.

A pilot study was conducted on a total of 39 participants. At the end of the first week, the participants had an increase in muscle mass and also lost 7 pounds on average. Research has proven that in this initial week, the weight loss that is witnessed is mostly from water, glycogen, and muscle, and only one-third of it is from fat (Manfred J. Müller, 2016). The major sirtfoods include red wine, kale, soy, strawberries, matcha green tea, extra virgin olive oil, walnuts, buckwheat, capers, lovage, coffee, dark chocolate, Medjool dates, turmeric, red chicory, parsley, onions, arugula, and blueberries (Kathrin Pallauf, 2013).

Chapter 2: Sirtfood Juice Recipes

Green Juice

Total Prep & Cooking Time: Five minutes

Yields: 1 serving

Nutrition Facts: Calories: 182.3 | Carbs: 42.9g | Protein: 6g | Fat: 1.5g | Fiber: 12.7g

Ingredients:

- Half a green apple
- Two sticks of celery
- Five grams of parsley
- Thirty grams of rocket
- Seventy-five grams of kale
- Half a teaspoon of matcha green tea
- Juice of half a lemon
- One cm of ginger

Method:

1. Juice the kale, rocket, celery sticks, green apple, and parsley in a juicer.

2. Add the lemon juice into the green juice by squeezing it with your hand.

3. Take a glass and pour a little amount of the green juice into it. Add the matcha green tea and stir it in. Then, pour the remaining green juice into the glass and stir to combine everything properly.

4. You can choose to save it for later or drink it straight away.

Blueberry Kale Smoothie

Total Prep & Cooking Time: Five minutes

Yields: 1 serving

Nutrition Facts: Calories: 240 | Carbs: 37.9g | Protein: 17.2g | Fat: 3.6g | Fiber: 7g

Ingredients:

- Half a cup each of
  - Plain low-fat yogurt
  - Blueberries (frozen or fresh)
  - Kale, chopped
- Half a banana
- Half a teaspoon of cinnamon powder
- One tablespoon of flaxseed meal
- One scoop of protein powder
- Half a cup of water (optional)
- Two handfuls of ice (you can add more if you like)

Method:

1. Take a high-speed blender and add all the ingredients in it.

2. Blend everything together until you get a smooth puree.

3. Pour the blueberry kale smoothie in a glass and serve cold.

Tropical Kale Smoothie

Total Prep & Cooking Time: 10 minutes

Yields: 2 servings

Nutrition Facts: Calories: 187 | Carbs: 46.8g | Protein: 3.5g | Fat: 0.5g | Fiber: 4.7g

Ingredients:

- Half a cup to one cup of orange juice (about 120 ml to 240 ml)
- One banana, chopped (use frozen banana, is possible)
- Two cups of pineapple (about 330 grams), chopped (use frozen pineapple if possible)
- One and a half cups of kale (around 90 grams), chopped

Method:

1. Add the chopped bananas, pineapple, kale, and orange juice into a blender and blend everything together until you get a smooth puree.

2. You can add more orange juice if you need to attain a smoothie consistency. The amount of frozen fruit used directly affects the consistency of the smoothie.

3. Pour the smoothie equally into two glasses and serve cold.

Strawberry Oatmeal Smoothie

Total Prep & Cooking Time: 5 minutes

Yields: 2 servings

Nutrition Facts: Calories: 236.1 | Carbs: 44.9g | Protein: 7.6g | Fat: 3.7g | Fiber: 5.9g

Ingredients:

- Half a tsp. of vanilla extract
- Fourteen frozen strawberries
- One banana (cut into chunks)
- Half a cup of rolled oats
- One cup of soy milk
- One and a half tsps. of white sugar

Method:

1. Take a blender. Add the strawberries, banana, oats, and soy milk.

2. Then add sugar and vanilla extract.

3. Blend until the texture becomes smooth.

4. Then pour it into a glass and serve.

Chapter 3: Main Course Recipes for Sirtfood Diet

Green Juice Salad

Total Prep & Cooking Time: Ten minutes

Yields: 1 serving

Nutrition Facts: Calories: 199 | Carbs: 27g | Protein: 10g | Fat: 8.2g | Fiber: 9.2g

Ingredients:

- Six walnuts, halved

- Half of a green apple, sliced

- Two sticks of celery, sliced

- One tablespoon each of

  o Parsley

  o Olive oil

- One handful of rocket

- Two handfuls of kale, sliced

- One cm of ginger, grated

- Juice of half a lemon

- Salt and pepper to taste

Method:

1. To make the dressing, add the olive oil, ginger, lemon juice, salt, and pepper in a jam jar. Shake the jar to combine everything together.

2. Keep the sliced kale in a large bowl and add the dressing over it. Massage the dressing for about a minute to mix it with the kale properly.

3. Lastly, add the remaining ingredients (walnuts, sliced green apple, celery sticks, parsley, and rocket) into the bowl and combine everything thoroughly.

King Prawns and Buckwheat Noodles

Total Prep & Cooking Time: Twenty minutes

Yields: 4 servings

Nutrition Facts: Calories: 496 | Carbs: 53.2g | Protein: 22.2g | Fat: 17.6g | Fiber: 4.8g

Ingredients:

- 600 grams of king prawn
- 300 grams of soba or buckwheat noodles (using 100 percent buckwheat is recommended)
- One bird's eye chili, membranes, and seeds eliminated and finely chopped (and more according to taste)
- Three cloves of garlic, finely chopped or grated
- Three cm of ginger, grated
- 100 grams of green beans, chopped
- 100 grams of kale, roughly chopped
- Two celery sticks, sliced
- One red onion, thinly sliced
- Two tablespoons each of
  - Parsley, finely chopped (or lovage, if you have it)
  - Soy sauce or tamari (and extra for serving)
  - Extra virgin olive oil

Method:

1. Boil the buckwheat noodles for three to five minutes or until they are cooked according to your liking. Drain the water and then rinse the noodles in cold water. Drizzle some olive oil on the top and mix it with the noodles. Keep this mixture aside.

2. Prepare the remaining ingredients while the noodles are boiling.

3. Place a large frying pan or a wok over low heat and add a little olive oil into it. Then add the celery and red onions and fry them for about three minutes so that they get soft.

4. Then add the green beans and kale and increase the heat to medium-high. Fry them for about three minutes.

5. Decrease the heat again and then add the prawns, chili, ginger, and garlic into the pan. Fry for another two to three minutes so that the prawns get hot all the way through.

6. Lastly, add in the buckwheat noodles, soy sauce/tamari, and cook it for another minute so that the noodles get warm again.

7. Sprinkle some chopped parsley on the top as a garnish and serve hot.

Red Onion Dhal and Buckwheat

Total Prep & Cooking Time: Thirty minutes

Yields: 4 servings

Nutrition Facts: Calories: 154 | Carbs: 9g | Protein: 19g | Fat: 2g | Fiber: 12g

Ingredients:

- 160 grams of buckwheat or brown rice
- 100 grams of kale (spinach would also be a good alternative)
- 200 ml of water
- 400 ml of coconut milk
- 160 grams of red lentils
- Two teaspoons each of
  - Garam masala
  - Turmeric
- One bird's eye chili, deseeded and finely chopped (plus more if you want it extra hot)
- Two cms of ginger, grated
- Three cloves of garlic, crushed or grated
- One red onion (small), sliced
- One tablespoon of olive oil

Method:

1. Take a large, deep saucepan and add the olive oil in it. Add the sliced onion and cook it on low heat with the lid closed for about five minutes so that they get softened.

2. Add the chili, ginger, and garlic and cook it for another minute.

3. Add a splash of water along with the garam masala and turmeric and cook for another minute.

4. Next add the coconut milk, red lentils along with 200 ml of water. You can do this by filling the can of coconut milk halfway with water and adding it into the saucepan.

5. Combine everything together properly and let it cook over low heat for about twenty minutes. Keep the lid on and keep stirring occasionally. If the dhal starts to stick to the pan, add a little more water to it.

6. Add the kale after twenty minutes and stir properly and put the lid back on. Let it cook for another five minutes. (If you're using spinach instead, cook for an additional one to two minutes)

7. Add the buckwheat in a medium-sized saucepan about fifteen minutes before the curry is cooked.

8. Add lots of boiling water into the buckwheat and boil the water again—Cook for about ten minutes. If you prefer softer buckwheat, you can cook it for a little longer.

9. Drain the buckwheat using a sieve and serve along with the dhal.

Chicken Curry

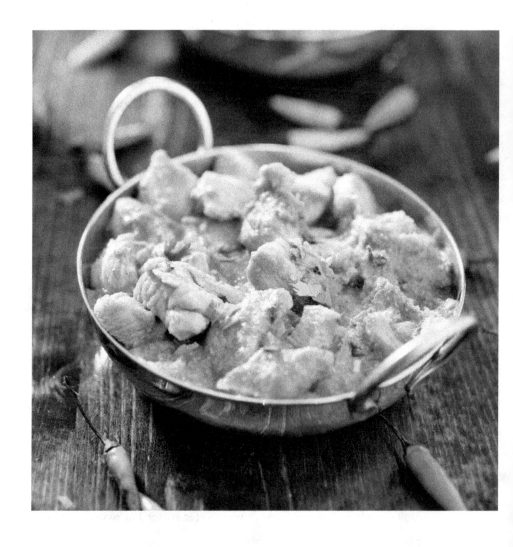

Total Prep & Cooking Time: 45 minutes

Yields: 4 servings

Nutrition Facts: Calories: 243 | Carbs: 7.5g | Protein: 28g | Fat: 11g | Fiber: 1.5g

Ingredients:

- 200 grams of buckwheat (you can also use basmati rice or brown rice)
- One 400ml tin of coconut milk
- Eight skinless and boneless chicken thighs, sliced into bite-sized chunks (you can also use four chicken breasts)
- One tablespoon of olive oil
- Six cardamom pods (optional)
- One cinnamon stick (optional)
- Two teaspoons each of
  - Ground turmeric
  - Ground cumin
  - Garam masala
- Two cm. of fresh ginger, peeled and coarsely chopped
- Three cloves of garlic, roughly chopped
- One red onion, roughly chopped
- Two tablespoons of freshly chopped coriander (and more for garnishing)

Method:

1. Add the ginger, garlic, and onions in a food processor and blitz to get a paste. You can also use a hand blender to make the paste. If you have neither, just finely chop the three ingredients and continue the following steps.

121

2. Add the turmeric powder, cumin, and garam masala into the paste and combine them together. Keep the paste aside.

3. Take a wide, deep pan (preferably a non-stick pan) and add one tablespoon of olive oil into it. Heat it over high heat for about a minute and then add the pieces of boneless chicken thighs. Increase the heat and stir-fry the chicken thighs for about two minutes. Then, reduce the heat and add the curry paste. Let the chicken cook in the curry paste for about three minutes and then pour half of the coconut milk (about 200ml) into it. You can also add the cardamom and cinnamon if you're using them.

4. Let it boil for some time and then reduce the heat and let it simmer for thirty minutes. The curry sauce will get thick and delicious.

5. You can add a splash of coconut milk if your curry sauce begins to get dry. You might not need to add extra coconut milk at all, but you can add it if you want a slightly more saucy curry.

6. Prepare your side dishes and other accompaniments (buckwheat or rice) while the curry is cooking.

7. Add the chopped coriander as a garnish when the curry is ready and serve immediately with the buckwheat or rice.

Chickpea Stew With Baked Potatoes

Total Prep & Cooking Time: One hour and ten minutes

Yields: 4 to 6 servings

Nutrition Facts: Calories: 348.3 | Carbs: 41.2g | Protein: 7.2g | Fat: 16.5g | Fiber: 5.3g

Ingredients:

- Two yellow peppers, chopped into bite-sized pieces (you can also use other colored bell peppers)
- Two 400-grams tins each of
  - Chickpeas (you can also use kidney beans) (don't drain the water if you prefer including it)
  - Chopped tomatoes
- Two cm. of ginger, grated
- Four cloves of garlic, crushed or grated
- Two red onions, finely chopped
- Four to six potatoes, prickled all over
- Two tablespoons each of
  - Turmeric
  - Cumin seeds
  - Olive oil
  - Unsweetened cocoa powder (or cacao, if you want)
  - Parsley (and extra for garnishing)

- Half a teaspoon to two teaspoons of chili flakes (you can add according to how hot you like things)
- A splash of water
- Side salad (optional)
- Salt and pepper according to your taste (optional)

Method:

1. Preheat your oven to 200 degrees Celsius.

2. In the meantime, prepare all the other ingredients.

3. Place your baking potatoes in the oven when it gets hot enough and allow it to cook for an hour so that they are cooked according to your preference. You can also use your regular method to bake the potatoes if it's different from this method.

4. When the potatoes are cooking in the oven, place a large wide saucepan over low heat and add the olive oil along with the chopped red onion into it. Keep the lid on and let the onions cook for five minutes. The onions should turn soft but shouldn't turn brown.

5. Take the lid off and add the chili, cumin, ginger, and garlic into the saucepan. Let it cook on low heat for another minute and then add the turmeric along with a tiny splash of water and cook it for a further minute. Make sure that the pan does not get too dry.

6. Then, add in the yellow pepper, canned chickpeas (along with the chickpea liquid), cacao or cocoa powder, and chopped tomatoes. Bring

the mixture to a boil and then let it simmer on low heat for about forty-five minutes so that the sauce gets thick and unctuous (make sure that it doesn't burn). The stew and the potatoes should complete cooking at roughly the same time.

7. Finally, add some salt and pepper as per your taste along with the parsley and stir them in the stew.

8. You can add the stew on top of the baked potatoes and serve. You can also serve the stew with a simple side salad.

Blueberry Pancakes

Total Prep & Cooking Time: 25 minutes

Yields: 2 servings

Nutrition Facts: Calories: 84 | Carbs: 11g | Protein: 2.3g | Fat: 3.5g | Fiber: 0g

Ingredients:

- 225 grams of blueberries
- 150 grams of rolled oats
- Six eggs
- Six bananas
- One-fourth of a teaspoon of salt
- Two teaspoons of baking powder

Method:

1. Add the rolled oats in a high-speed blender and pulse it for about a minute or so to get the oat flour. Before adding the oats to the blender, make sure that it is very dry. Otherwise, your oat flour will turn soggy.

2. Then, add the eggs and bananas along with the salt and baking soda into the blender and blend them together for another two minutes until you get a smooth batter.

3. Take a large bowl and transfer the mixture into it. Then add the blueberries and fold them into the mixture. Let it rest for about ten minutes to allow the baking powder to activate.

4. To make the pancakes, place a frying pan on medium-high heat and add a dollop of butter into it. The butter will help to make your pancakes really crispy and delicious.

5. Add a few spoonfuls of the blueberry pancake batter into the frying pan and cook it until the bottom side turns golden. Once the bottom turns golden, toss the pancake and fry the other side.

6. Serve them hot and enjoy.

Sirtfood Bites

Total Prep & Cooking Time: 1 hour + 15 minutes

Yields: 15-20 bites

Nutrition Facts: Calories: 58.1 | Carbs: 10.1g | Protein: 0.9g | Fat: 2.3g | Fiber: 1.2g

Ingredients:

- One tablespoon each of
  - o   Extra virgin olive oil
  - o   Ground turmeric
  - o   Cocoa powder
- Nine ounces of Medjool dates, pitted (about 250 grams)
- One ounce (about thirty grams) of dark chocolate (85% cocoa solids), break them into pieces (you can also use one-fourth of a cup of cocoa nibs)
- One teaspoon of vanilla extract (you can also take the scraped seeds of one vanilla pod)
- One cup of walnuts (about 120 grams)
- One to two tablespoons of water

Method:

1. Add the chocolate and walnuts in a food processor and blitz them until you get a fine powder.

2. Add the Medjool dates, cocoa powder, ground turmeric, extra-virgin olive oil, and vanilla extract into the food processor and blend them together until the mixture forms a ball. Depending on the consistency of the mixture, you can choose to add or skip the water. Make sure that the mixture is not too sticky.

3. Make bite-sized balls from the mixture using your hands and keep them in the refrigerator in an airtight container. Refrigerate them for at least an hour before consuming them.

4. To get a finish of your liking, you can roll the balls in some more dried coconut or cocoa. You can store the balls in the refrigerator for up to a week.

Flank Steak With Broccoli Cauliflower Gratin

Total Prep & Cooking Time: 55 minutes

Yields: 4 servings

Nutrition Facts: Calories: 839 | Carbs: 8g | Protein: 43g | Fat: 70g | Fiber: 3g

Ingredients:

- Two tablespoons of olive oil
- Twenty ounces of flank steak
- One-fourth teaspoon salt
- Four ounces of divided shredded cheese
- Half cup of heavy whipping cream
- Eight ounces of cauliflower
- Eight ounces of broccoli
- Salt and pepper

For the pepper sauce,

- One tablespoon soy sauce
- One and a half cups of heavy whipping cream
- Half teaspoon ground black pepper

For the garnishing,

- Two tablespoons of freshly chopped parsley

Method:

1. At first, you have to preheat your oven to four hundred degrees Fahrenheit. Then you need to apply butter on a baking dish (eight by eight inches).

2. Then you have to clean and then trim the cauliflower and broccoli. Then you need to cut them into florets, and their stem needs to be sliced.

3. Then you have to boil the broccoli and cauliflower for about five minutes in salted water.

4. After boiling, you need to drain out all the water and keep the vegetables aside. Then you have to take a saucepan over medium heat and add half portion of the shredded cheese, heavy cream, and salt. Then you need to whisk them together until the cheese gets melted. Then you have to add the cauliflower and the broccoli and mix them in.

5. Place the cauliflower and broccoli mixture in a baking dish. Then you have to take the rest half portion of the cheese and add—Bake for about twenty minutes in the oven.

6. Season with salt and pepper on both sides of the meat.

7. Then you have to take a large frying pan over medium-high heat and fry the meat for about four to five minutes on each side.

8. After that, take a cutting board and place the meat on it. Then you have to leave the meat for about ten to fifteen minutes before you start to slice it.

9. Take the frying pan, and in it, you need to pour soy sauce, cream, and pepper. Then you have to bring it to a boil and allow the sauce to simmer until the sauce becomes creamy in texture. Then you need to taste it and then season it with some more salt and pepper according to your taste.

Kale Celery Salad

Total Prep & Cooking Time: 15 minutes

Yields: 4 servings

Nutrition Facts: 196 | Carbs: 20g | Protein: 5.7g | Fat: 11.5g | Fiber: 4.8g

Ingredients:

- Half a cup of crumbled feta cheese
- Half a cup of chopped and toasted walnuts
- One wedge lemon
- One red apple, crisp
- Two celery stalks
- Eight dates, pitted dried
- Four cups of washed and dried baby kale (stemmed)

For the dressing,

- Three tbsps. olive oil
- One tsp. maple syrup (or you can use any other sweetener as per your preference)
- Four tsps. balsamic vinegar
- Freshly ground salt and black pepper

Method:

1. At first, you have to take a platter or a wide serving bowl. Then you need to place the baby kale in it.

2. Cut the dates into very thin slices, lengthwise. Then you need to place it in another small bowl.

3. After that, you have to peel the celery and then cut them into halves, lengthwise.

4. Then you need to take your knife, hold it in a diagonal angle, and then cut the celery into thin pieces (approximately one to two inches each). Add these pieces to the dates.

5. Then you have to cut the sides off the apple. You need to cut very thin slices from those pieces.

6. Over the apple slices, you need to put some lemon juice to prevent them from browning.

7. For preparing the dressing, you have to take a small bowl, add maple syrup, olive oil, and vinegar. Then you need to whisk them together.

8. Once done, you have to season with freshly ground pepper and two pinches of salt.

9. Before serving, you need to take most of the dressing and pour it over the salad. Then you have to toss nicely so that they get combined. Then you need to pour the rest of the portion of the dressing over the dates and celery.

10. On the top, you have to add the date mixture, feta cheese, apple slices, and walnuts.

Buckwheat Stir Fry

Total Prep & Cooking Time: 28 minutes

Yields: 8 servings

Nutrition Facts: Calories: 258 | Carbs: 35.1g | Protein: 6.8g | Fat: 11.9g | Fiber: 2g

Ingredients:

For the buckwheat,

- Three cups of water
- One and a half cups of uncooked roasted buckwheat groats
- Pinch of salt

For the stir fry,

- Half a cup of finely chopped basil
- Half a cup of finely chopped parsley
- One teaspoon salt
- Four tablespoons of divided red palm oil or coconut oil
- Two cups of drained and chopped marinated artichoke hearts
- Four large bell peppers (sliced into strips)
- Four large minced cloves of garlic
- One bunch of finely chopped kale (ribs removed)

Method:

For making the buckwheat,

1. In a medium-sized pot, pour the buckwheat. Then rinse with cold water and drain the water. Repeat this process for about two to three times.

2. Then add three cups of water to it and also add a pinch of salt. Cover the pot and bring it to a boil.

3. Reduce the heat to low and then cook for about fifteen minutes. Keep the lid on and remove the pot from the heat.

4. Leave it for three minutes and then fluff with a fork.

For making the stir fry,

1. At first, you have to take a ceramic non-stick wok and preheat over medium heat. Then you need to add one tablespoon of oil and coat it. Then you have to add garlic and then sauté for about ten seconds. Then you need to add kale and then add one-fourth teaspoon of salt. Then you need to sauté it accompanied by occasional stirring, until it shrinks in half. Then you have to transfer it to a medium-sized bowl.

2. Then again return to the wok, turn the heat on high, and pour one tablespoon of oil. You need to add one-fourth teaspoon salt and pepper. Then you have to sauté it until it turns golden brown in color. Once done, you need to place it in the bowl containing kale.

3. Then you have to reduce the heat to low, and you need to add two tablespoons of oil. Add the cooked buckwheat and stir it nicely so that it gets coated in the oil. Then after turning off the heat, you need to add the kale and peppers, basil, parsley, artichoke hearts, and half teaspoon salt. Gently stir and serve it hot.

Kale Omelet

Total Prep & Cooking Time: 10 minutes

Yields: 1 serving

Nutrition Facts: Calories: 339 | Carbs: 8.6g | Protein: 15g | Fat: 28.1g | Fiber: 4.4g

Ingredients:

- One-fourth sliced avocado
- Pinch of red pepper (crushed)
- One tsp. sunflower seeds (unsalted)
- One tbsp. of freshly chopped cilantro
- One tbsp. lime juice
- One cup of chopped kale
- Two tsps. of extra-virgin olive oil
- One tsp. of low-fat milk
- Two eggs
- Salt

Method:

1. At first, take a small bowl and pour milk. Then you have to add the eggs and salt to it. Beat the mixture thoroughly. Then take a small non-stick skillet over medium heat, and add one tsp. of oil and heat it. Then add the egg mixture and cook for about one to two minutes, until the time you notice that the center is still a bit runny, but the bottom has become set. Then you need to flip the omelet and cook the other side for another thirty seconds until it is set too. One done, transfer the omelet to a plate.

2. Toss the kale with one tsp. of oil, sunflower seeds, cilantro, lime juice, salt, and crushed red pepper in another bowl. Then return to the omelet on the plate and top it off with avocado and the kale salad.

Tuna Rocket Salad

Total Prep & Cooking Time: 20 minutes

Yields: 4 servings

Nutrition Facts: Calories: 321 | Carbs: 20g | Protein: 33g | Fat: 12g | Fiber: 9.5g

Ingredients:

- Twelve leaves of basil (fresh)

- Two bunches of washed and dried rocket (trimmed)

- One and a half tbsps. of olive oil

- Freshly ground black pepper and salt

- Sixty grams of kalamata olives cut into halves, lengthwise (drained pitted)

- One thinly sliced and halved red onion

- Two coarsely chopped ripe tomatoes

- Four hundred grams of rinsed and drained cannellini beans

- Four hundred grams of drained tuna

- 2 cm cubes of one multigrain bread roll

Method:

1. At first, you need to preheat your oven to 200 degrees Celsius.

2. After that, take a baking tray and line it with a foil.

3. Then you have to spread the cubes of bread over the baking tray evenly.

4. Put the baking tray inside the oven and cook it for about ten minutes until it turns golden in color.

5. In the meantime, you have to take a large bowl and add the olives, onions, tomatoes, cannellini beans, and tuna. Then you need to season it with pepper and salt. Add some oil and then toss for smooth combining.

6. Your next step is to add the basil leaves, croutons, and the rocket. Then you need to toss gently to combine. After that, you can divide the salad into the serving bowls and serve.

Turmeric Baked Salmon

Total Prep & Cooking Time: 30 minutes

Yields: 4 servings

Nutrition Facts: Calories: 448 | Carbs: 2g | Protein: 34g | Fat: 33g | Fiber: 0.2g

Ingredients:

- One ripe yellow lemon
- Half a teaspoon of salt
- One teaspoon turmeric
- One tablespoon of dried thyme
- Half a cup of frozen, salted butter (you may require some more for greasing the pan)
- Four fresh one and a half inches thick salmon fillets (skin-on)

Method:

1. At first, you need to preheat your oven to 400 degrees Fahrenheit. Then with a thin layer of butter, you need to grease the bottom of the baking sheet. Rinse the salmon fillets and pat them dry. Then you have to place the salmon fillets on the buttered baking dish keeping the skin side down.

2. Take the lemons and cut them into four round slices. Remove the seeds and then cut each slice into two halves. Then you will have eight pieces.

3. Take a small dish and combine turmeric, dried thyme, and salt. Then you need to mix them well until they are nicely combined. On the top of the salmon fillets, you need to evenly sprinkle the spice mixture.

4. Place two lemon slices over each salmon fillet.

5. After that, you need to grate the cold butter on the top of the salmon fillets evenly. Allow the butter to meltdown and form a delicious sauce.

6. Then you have to cover the pan with parchment or aluminum foil. Put it inside the oven and cook for about fifteen to twenty minutes according to your desire. The cooking time is dependent on the thickness of the salmon fillets. You can check whether it is done or not by cutting into the center.

7. Once done, remove it from the oven and then uncover it. The butter sauce needs to be spooned over from the tray.

8. Top it off with fresh mint and serve.

Chapter 4: One-Week Meal Plan

Day 1

8 AM – Green Juice

12 PM - Blueberry Kale Smoothie

4 PM – Tropical Kale Smoothie

8 PM – Turmeric Baked Salmon

Day 2

8 AM – Tropical Kale Smoothie

12 PM – Green Juice

4 PM – Strawberry Oatmeal Smoothie

8 PM – King Prawns and Buckwheat Noodles

Day 3

8 AM – Strawberry Oatmeal Smoothie

12 PM – Tropical Kale Smoothie

4 PM – Green Juice

8 PM – Buckwheat Stir Fry

Day 4

8 AM – Blueberry Kale Smoothie

12 PM – Green Juice

4 PM – Green Juice Salad

8 PM – Tuna Rocket Salad

Day 5

8 AM – Green Juice

12 PM – Tropical Kale Smoothie

4 PM – Sirtfood Bites

8 PM – Chicken Curry

Day 6

8 AM – Strawberry Oatmeal Smoothie

12 PM – Green Juice

4 PM – Kale Celery Salad

8 PM – Flank Steak with Broccoli Cauliflower Gratin

Day 7

8 AM – Tropical Kale Smoothie

12 PM – Blueberry Kale Smoothie

4 PM – Kale Omelet

8 PM – Chickpea Stew with Baked Potatoes

PART IV

PCOS is now a growing problem among women, and in this chapter, we are going to discuss a special diet that is going to help you get past it.

Chapter 1: What Is PCOS?

Quite a lot of you might have come across the term 'PCOS.' Polycystic ovary syndrome or polycystic ovarian syndrome is a very common hormonal disorder that is known to affect women aged 15 to 44 years, i.e., child-bearing years. Reliable studies state that nearly 2.2 to 26.7% of women of the above-mentioned age group suffer from PCOS. This condition affects the hormone level of a woman. Such a condition might affect your fertility. In women, PCOS is the most general cause of infertility. You might skip your menstrual period for such hormone imbalance. Moreover, getting pregnant becomes harder for those women who are going through such health conditions.

Usually, women who suffer from PCOS might face prolonged or infrequent menstrual periods. In some cases, predicting the exact date of periods becomes difficult. If you have PCOS, then the hormones of reproduction are not in balance. Hormones such as progesterone and estrogen that are produced in the ovaries regulate a woman's menstrual cycle. PCOS directly affects the ovaries as well as ovulation. Besides these two hormones, your ovaries even produce male hormones or androgens. Individuals with PCOS have a tendency to produce excessive amounts of male hormones. Many tiny sacs filled with fluids called cysts tend to develop in the ovaries of some women having PCOS. But, not everyone who is suffering from this syndrome has multiple cysts in their ovaries.

Polycystic ovary syndrome also causes the growth of unwanted facial and body hair. Excess androgen secretion even causes acne as well as hair loss, which might further lead to baldness of male pattern. Your skin might become oilier and lead to breakouts on specific areas like the chest, upper back, and face. Numerous reports state that approximately 80% of those women suffering from PCOS are either obese or overweight. Obesity worsens the complications related to this disorder. Heavier bleeding than usual is also another common symptom of this syndrome. Hormonal changes or imbalance also trigger headaches in many women. Mood swings or frequent mood changes are also a sign of the polycystic ovarian syndrome. In some instances, skin gets darkened, or dark patches can be seen under the breasts. These patches can also appear on the neck region, and also in the armpit.

Not only does this hormonal condition affects your fertility, but it also increases the risk of various health problems such as high blood pressure, heart disease, stroke, type 2 diabetes, endometrial cancer, etc. Various other complications include anxiety, depression, sleep apnea, eating disorders, gestational diabetes, non-alcoholic steatohepatitis, etc. An interesting fact is that the maximum number of women don't even know that they have PCOS. A study stated that nearly 70% of women having PCOS have not yet been diagnosed.

The treatment of PCOS varies from person to person, depending on the symptoms and other health complications. Once it is diagnosed, its treatment begins with changes in lifestyle such as regular exercise, prescribed diet plan, weight loss, etc. If a nutritious diet is combined with daily workout, then it is highly beneficial. For those who are overweight, shedding just 5-10% of extra pounds might prove helpful in improving the other symptoms.

Chapter 2: Vegetarian Recipes

Read on to find out some delicious recipes that you can include in your PCOS diet.

Breakfast Yogurt Parfait
Total Prep & Cooking Time: 10 minutes

Yields: One glass

Nutrition Facts: Calories: 238 | Carbs: 10g | Protein: 14g | Fat: 17g | Fiber: 3g

Ingredients:

- Two tbsps. of mixed nuts (the nuts should be raw and chopped into pieces)
- One yogurt (two good from peach or strawberry)
- A quarter cup of berries (fresh)

Method:

1. Take a bowl and form layers of chopped nuts and then the second layer of berries and the third layer with yogurt. You can add fixings into the cup of yogurt.

2. Enjoy the yogurt parfait immediately.

Notes: *If you are using toasted nuts, you can brush them with few drops of avocado oil and then season with some salt and sweetener. Toss the ingredients well to incorporate and then bake for eight minutes at a temperature of 325 degrees F.*

Banana Pancakes

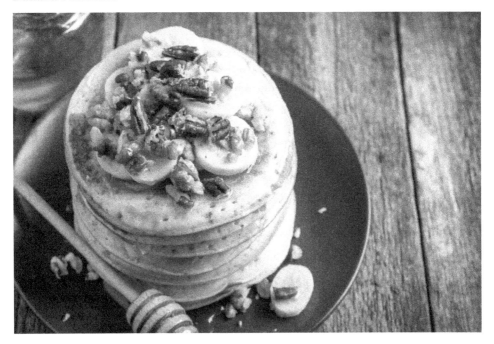

Total Prep & Cooking Time: 15 minutes

Yields: Two servings

Nutrition facts: Calories: 124 | Carbs: 13.8g | Protein: 6.9g | Fat: 4.9g | Fiber: 1.5g

Ingredients:

- One medium-sized banana
- Two eggs (large-sized)

Method:

1. Process the banana and the eggs in a blender to form a smooth puree.

2. Place a skillet over a medium flame and pour one to two drops of oil. For each pancake, you will require only two tablespoons of the egg-banana batter. With this calculation, you can put about four mounds of the dough into the skillet—Cook the pancakes for four minutes, allowing the edges to brown.

3. Flip the pancakes and cook for about two minutes again. Transfer to a serving plate. Repeat the same procedure with the remaining batter.

4. Serve and enjoy the delicious banana pancakes.

Notes: You can coat the skillet with oil using a piece of a paper towel. Crumble the paper towel and slowly dab on the bottom of the skillet.

Mushroom and Asparagus Frittata

Total Prep & Cooking Time: 45 minutes

Yields: Eight servings

Nutrition Facts: Calories: 130 | carbs: 5g | Protein: 9g | Fat: 8g | Fiber: 1g

Ingredients:

- Eight eggs (large-sized)
- Two tbsps. of lemon juice
- A quarter tsp. of pepper
- Eight oz. of asparagus spears (frozen and thawed)
- Half a cup each of
- Pepper, green or red (chopped finely)
- Ricotta cheese (whole-milk)
- Half a tsp. of salt
- One tbsp. of olive oil
- One large-sized onion (thinly sliced and halved)
- A quarter cup of sliced mushrooms (baby Portobello)

Method:

1. Set the oven at a temperature of 350 degrees F.

2. Take a bowl and add the cheese, pepper, juice, egg, and salt. Whisk all the ingredients properly.

3. Place a ten-inch skillet on the oven and turn the flame to moderate heat. The skillet must be ovenproof. To the skillet, add the pepper, asparagus, mushrooms, and onion. Cook for eight minutes until the pepper and onion are tender.

4. First, you will have to remove the skillet from the heat. Then you can remove the asparagus from the skillet. Reserve eight spears of the asparagus and cut the rest into the size of two inches. Return the sliced asparagus into the skillet and put the skillet back on the oven. Stir in the egg mixture. Arrange the reserved spears of asparagus on the egg mixture so that it looks like wheel spokes.

5. Bake the mixture for twenty-five minutes. Let it stand for five minutes.

6. Cut the preparation into wedges.

Strawberry Salad

Total Prep & Cooking Time: 30 minutes

Yields: Ten servings

Nutrition Facts: Calories: 110 | Carbs: 13g | Protein: 2g | Fat: 6g | Fiber: 2g

Ingredients:

- A quarter cup each of

  o Sugar

  o Mayonnaise

- One bunch of torn romaine (approximately eight cups)

- Two cups of strawberries (fresh and halved)

- One small-sized onion, cut into half and thinly sliced

- One tbsp. each of

  o Two percent milk

  o Sour cream

- One and a half tsps. of poppy seeds

- A one-third cup of almonds (silvered)

- Two tbsps. of sugar

- Two and a quarter tsps. of vinegar (cider)

Method:

1. Place a small yet heavy skillet over moderate flame. To the skillet, add the sugar and cook for about ten minutes until it melts into a caramel-colored substance. Stir in the almonds until they get coated with the melted sugar. Transfer the content to a foil and spread them evenly to cool.

2. Take a bowl and add strawberries, romaine, and onion to it. Whisk the contents required for the dressing and toss in the salad. Break the almonds into pieces and then spread them over the salad in the bowl.

3. Serve them immediately.

Low Carb Green Smoothie

Total Prep & Cooking Time: 5 minutes

Yields: Two glasses of smoothie

Nutrition Facts: Calories: 168 | Carbs: 4.8g | Protein: 6g | Fat: 4g | Fiber: 7g

Ingredients:

- One medium-sized avocado (pitted and peeled)
- One and a half cups of coconut milk (unsweetened)
- One tablespoon each of
  - Powdered peanut butter
  - Lemon juice (freshly squeezed)
- One cup of spinach
- One spoonful of protein powder (vanilla flavored and sugar-free)

Method:

1. You will require a blender for preparing this smoothie. Add all the ingredients to it and process it for about thirty seconds. It will form a smooth puree.

2. You can taste the puree and adjust the taste by adding any component you think is less.

3. Pour in two tall glasses and enjoy.

Peanut Butter Balls

Total Prep & Cooking Time: 20 minutes

Yields: Eighteen balls

Nutrition Facts: Calories: 194 | Carbs: 7g | Protein: 7g | Fat: 17g | Fiber: 3g

Ingredients:

- One cup each of
  - Peanuts (chopped finely and salted)
  - Sweetener (powdered)
  - Peanut butter
- Chocolate chips (eight ounces)

Method:

1. Combine the sweetener, chopped peanuts, and the peanut butter to form a dough. Make eighteen small and round balls with the dough. Take a baking sheet and line it with wax paper.

2. Arrange the balls on the sheet in rows.

3. Insert chocolate chips in the microwave to melt them.

4. Dip the peanut balls in chocolate one by one and return them to the sheet.

5. Place the balls inside the refrigerator until the chocolate completely sets.

Low Carb Cheesecake

Total Prep & Cooking Time: 1 hour 10 minutes

Yields: Twelve cheesecakes

Nutrition Facts: Calories: 600 | Carbs: 7g | Protein: 14g | Fat: 54g | Fiber: 2g

Ingredients:

For preparing the crust,

- One and a half cups of almond flour
- One tsp. of cinnamon
- A quarter cup of sweetener (powdered)
- Six tbsps. of melted butter

For preparing the filling,

- Eight oz. of cream cheese (full-fat), approximately six packages
- Five large-sized eggs kept at room temperature
- One tbsp. of vanilla extract
- Two cups of sweetener (powdered)
- Eight oz. of sour cream (at room temperature)

Method:

1. Set the temperature of the oven at 325 degrees F. Place the rack at the center of the oven.

2. Take a medium-sized bowl and add the ingredients for preparing the crust as listed above. Add butter to the bowl. Combine them well.

3. For making these cheesecakes, you will require a pan of dimension 10-inch x 4-inch. Pour crust mixture into the pan and press the mixture to

the pan's bottom with a flattened cup. Put mixture into the refrigerator for about twenty minutes.

4. Take a small bowl and then pour the cream cheese into it. Beat the cream with a hand mixer into a fluffy mixture with a light consistency.

5. Add sweetener (one-third) at first and continue beating with the hand mixer.

6. To the mixture, add eggs and then beat until the mixture becomes completely incorporated.

7. Finally, add in vanilla and sour cream and combine well.

8. Fill the crust with the cheesecake mixture and pour some of it on the outer surface as well. Bake the dough for about fifty minutes. The cake should have a jiggly center, and the upper part should be opaque.

9. Turn off the oven but allow the cheesecake to stay in there for thirty minutes.

10. Take out the pan and insert a knife in the cake to check if the cake stick or not. Leave the cake for one hour on the countertop.

11. Cover the pan with a plastic wrapper and then refrigerate for eight hours.

12. After the said time, remove the cake from the pan, slice it into twelve pieces, and decorate the top and serve.

Tropical Smoothie Bowl

Total Prep & Cooking Time: 5 minutes

Yields: 2 servings

Nutrition Facts: Calories: 180 | Carbs: 43g | Protein: 3g | Fat: 2g | Fiber: 5g

Ingredients:

- One cup each of
  - Almond milk
  - Frozen pineapple chunks
  - Frozen mango chunks
- One frozen banana, sliced

Method:

1. Add the pineapple, mango, and banana in a blender along with the almond milk and pulse them together for a few minutes, stopping and occasionally stirring until it gets smooth but still thick. You can add some more liquid if required.

2. Pour the smoothie equally into two separate bowls. Add any desired topping and serve cold.

Chapter 3: Non-Vegetarian Recipes

Broccoli and Bacon Egg Burrito

Total Prep & Cooking Time: 20 minutes

Yields: One serving

Nutrition facts: Calories: 259 | Carbs: 9.8g | Protein: 15.4g | Fat: 5.9g | Fiber: 3.3g

Ingredients:

- One slice of bacon
- A quarter cup of tomato (chopped)
- One tbsp. of milk (reduced-fat)
- One cup of broccoli (chopped)
- One egg (large)
- One scallion (chopped)
- One tsp. of canola or avocado oil
- One-eighth tsp. each of
  - Pepper (ground)
  - Salt
- Two tbsps. of cheddar cheese (sharp and shredded)

Method:

1. Cook the bacon for six minutes in a medium-sized skillet, putting the flame to moderate heat. Flip them twice while cooking to give them a crisp. Remove bacon to another plate that is lined with a paper towel.

2. Maintaining the temperature, put the broccoli pieces to the skillet, and then cook. Stir them for three minutes until they become soft. Add the chopped tomatoes and stir everything. Transfer to a bowl and keep aside.

3. In the meantime, take a bowl and place the egg, scallion, pepper, milk, and salt. Whisk them properly. Wash the skillet after cooking the vegetables and oil to it. Turn the flame to moderate heat and then add egg mixture to the boiling oil. Tilt the pan right and left to allow the mix to make a coating at the bottom and then cook the mixture for about two minutes without disturbing it.

4. Flip the egg mixture with a spatula (made of silicone, and it should be thin and full). Cook the mixture with sprinkled cheese for a minute and then allow the preparation to set completely.

5. Transfer to a serving plate. Stuff the lower part of the tortilla with broccoli mixture and the upper part with the bacon. Roll the preparation to form a burrito and enjoy it.

Smoked Salmon and Avocado Omelet

Total Prep & Cooking Time: 10 minutes

Yields: One serving

Nutrition Facts: Calories: 323 | Carbs: 5.3g | Protein: 19g | Fat: 5.5g | Fiber: 3.4g

Ingredients:

- Two eggs (large-sized)
- To taste: Salt
- A quarter-sized avocado (chopped)
- One tbsp. of fresh basil (chopped)
- One tsp. of milk (low-fat)
- One and a half tsp. of olive oil (extra-virgin, divided)
- One oz. of salmon (smoked)

Method:

1. Take a bowl and then beat the eggs into it. Add the milk and sprinkle salt to it. Whisk them properly.

2. Place a skillet (non-stick) on the oven, putting the flame to moderate heat. Add one tsp. of oil to the skillet and then add the egg mixture. Cook the content so that they set with a slightly runny center. It will take you two minutes and not more.

3. Flip the omelet and cook this side for thirty seconds to place.

4. Transfer the preparation to a serving plate and top it with salmon, basil, and avocado. Drizzle the omelet with the remaining oil to enhance the taste.

BLT Chicken Salad

Total prep & Cooking Time: 20 minutes

Yields: Eight servings

Nutrition Facts: Calories: 281 | Carbs: 5g | Protein: 23g | Fat: 19g | Fiber: 2g

Ingredients:

- Half a cup of mayonnaise
- Two tbsps. of onion (finely chopped)
- A quarter tsp. of pepper
- Two large-sized tomatoes (chopped finely)
- One and a half lb. of chicken breasts, skinless and boneless (you must cook the chicken and cut it into small cubes)
- Two large-sized eggs, hard-boiled (slice them into halves)
- Three to four tbsps. of barbeque sauce
- One tbsp. of lemon juice
- Eight cups of salad greens (you must tear the leaves into small pieces)
- Ten strips of bacon (crumbled and cooked)

Method:

1. Take a small-sized bowl. To it, add the mayonnaise, chopped onion, pepper, sauce, and juice. Combine the mixture properly to incorporate the ingredients. Cover the bowl with a lid and keep it inside the refrigerator. Allow it to stay there until the time of serving.

2. Take another bowl, this time a large one. Place the salad greens in it. Spread the chicken cubes, bacon, and tomatoes on top. Garnish the bowl content with egg slices. Take out the dressing and drizzle it over the bowl.

3. Serve and enjoy!

Black Beans and Chicken Chili

Total Prep & Cooking Time: 35 minutes

Yields: Ten servings

Nutrition Facts: Calories: 236 | Carbs: 21g | Protein: 22g | Fat: 6g | Fiber: 6g

Ingredients:

- One three-fourth lb. of chicken breasts (skinless and boneless, cut into cubes)
- One large-sized onion (finely chopped)
- Four oz. of green chilies (chopped)
- Two tbsps. of chili powder
- One tsp. of coriander (ground)
- Twenty-eight oz. of sliced tomatoes (Italian and stewed)
- One cup of water
- Two medium-sized red peppers (sweet and chopped)
- Three tbsps. of olive oil
- Four cloves of garlic (diced)
- Two tsps. of cumin (ground)
- Two cans of drained and rinsed black beans
- One cup of beer or chicken broth

Method:

1. Pour few drops of oil in the Dutch oven. To the boiling oil, add the pepper, onions, and chicken. Cook until the chicken becomes brown and the onion becomes translucent. It will probably take you five minutes.

2. To the cooked chicken, add the garlic, cumin, coriander, chilies, and chili powder—Cook the whole preparation for an additional minute. Stir in tomatoes, half cup of water, beans, and the chicken broth. Cook until the water starts to boil and then reduce heat and then simmer. Stir occasionally for fifteen minutes. You may add some water if you like to have a watery consistency.

Cucumber Salmon Panzanella

Total Prep & Cooking Time: 20 minutes

Yields: Four servings

Nutrition Facts: Calories: 320 | Carbs: 13.8g | Protein: 26.4g | Fat: 2.8g | Fiber: 4.1g

Ingredients:

- Eight ounces of torn bread (country bread)
- Black pepper
- Three tablespoons of vinegar (red wine)
- Salt
- Two tablespoons of olive oil
- Four cucumbers (Persian)
- One teaspoon of caraway seeds
- One small-sized fennel bulb (chopped)
- Roasted salmon
- A quarter red onion, chopped
- One cup of arugula

Method:

1. Set the temperature of the oven at 425 degrees F.

2. Take a baking sheet (rimmed one is preferable). Add the olive oil, salt, pepper, and bread to the sheet and toss them well. Toast the sheet contents for ten minutes until browned and then set aside to cool.

3. Cut the cucumbers into half and then cut them crosswise with a knife.

4. Take a bowl and add red wine, caraway seeds, olive oil, and vinegar to it. Whisk them and then add the fennel bulb, cucumbers, red onion, and arugula to it. Stir well to combine.

5. Transfer to serving plates and top with flaked and roasted salmon and bread.

Rosemary-Lemon Chicken

Total Prep & Cooking Time: 55 minutes

Yields: Four servings

Nutrition facts: Calories: 289 | Carbs: 12g | Protein: 30g | Fat: 14g | Fiber: 4g

Ingredients:

- Two tablespoons of flat-leaf and fresh parsley (chopped)
- One large clove of garlic (minced)
- Three tablespoons of olive oil (extra-virgin)
- Black pepper (freshly ground)
- Two and a half pounds of chicken breasts (skin-on and bone-in)
- One onion, red (sliced into wedges of half-inch)
- One thinly sliced lemon
- One pound of broccoli
- Half teaspoon of red pepper (crushed)
- Kosher salt
- Two teaspoons of Dijon mustard
- One and a half tablespoons of rosemary (fresh and finely chopped)

Method:

1. Keep the oven preheated at a temperature of 425 degrees F.

2. Combine the rosemary, Dijon, garlic, one tbsp. of oil, and parsley in a pot. Season them with pepper and salt. Mix them well.

3. Line the chicken (underneath its skin) with the rosemary mixture and the lemon wedges (approximately eight). Rub the chicken surface with the rest of the rosemary mixture. Bake the rosemary-coated chicken for twenty-two minutes on a baking sheet.

4. In the meantime, take a bowl and add broccoli, red pepper, lemon wedges, two tbsp. of oil and onion to it. Sprinkle with pepper and salt. Toss them well.

5. Take the baking sheet out of the oven and arrange the chicken with the tossed vegetables all around. Again bake it for fourteen minutes.

6. Serve them on a plate and top with red pepper.

Zucchini Noodles and Turkey Meatballs

Total Prep & Cooking Time: 30 minutes

Yields: Four servings

Nutrition Facts: Calories: 526 | Crabs: 27g | Protein: 39g | Fat: 30g | Fiber: 6g

Ingredients:

- One pound of turkey (ground)
- One large-sized egg
- One and a half-ounce of grated parmesan cheese
- Kosher salt
- Two tablespoons of olive oil (extra-virgin)
- Four medium-sized zucchinis (sliced into noodle-like pieces)
- Black pepper (freshly ground)
- Twenty-five ounces of marinara sauce
- Four ounces of grated provolone cheese
- Two cloves of garlic (minced)
- A quarter cup of breadcrumbs (seasoned and dried)
- Three tablespoons of parsley (flat-leaf and fresh)

Method:

1. Add the breadcrumbs, parmesan, half tsp. each of pepper and salt, one clove of garlic, egg, turkey, and parsley in a bowl. Combine well and form twelve meatballs.

2. Heat one tbsp. of oil over a moderate flame in a skillet. Drop meatballs and then cook them, occasionally stirring for six minutes until browned. Reduce flame and add the marinara to the meatballs. Stir them occasionally to cook the meatballs thoroughly and thicken the sauce. You can cook for sixteen minutes or so. After they are done, transfer to another plate.

3. Add oil to the skillet keeping the flame to moderate heat. Then add the rest of the garlic pieces and the zucchini to the oil. Cook them for three minutes until the garlic is tenderized—season with pepper and salt.

4. Heat a grill over a high flame, keeping the rack on top. Sprinkle the meatballs with provolone and then place the balls over the rack. Broil for four minutes until browned.

5. Serve the meatballs with topped zucchini noodles and parmesan.

Cajun Shrimp Caesar Salad

Total Prep & Cooking Time: 15 minutes

Yields: Four servings

Nutrition Facts: Calories: 434 | Carbs: 12.7g | Protein: 29.5g | Fat: 30.6g | Fiber: 6.3g

Ingredients:

- Half a cup of salad dressing (Caesar)

- One tablespoon of Cajun seasoning

- Eight cups of romaine lettuce (finely chopped)

- Six tablespoons of shredded parmesan cheese

- One pound of shrimp (patted dry, peeled, and deveined)

- Two tablespoons of olive oil

- Two cups of diced Roma tomatoes

Method:

1. For the Caesar dressing- Combine one and a quarter cups of mayonnaise, two tablespoons each of Worcestershire sauce, lemon juice, and anchovy paste, six tablespoons of olive oil, salt, and pepper. Whisk them together to a small dough. Set the dressing aside.

2. Pour the Cajun seasoning in a bowl and add the shrimp pieces to it. Toss well to coat the shrimp with the seasoning.

3. Pour olive oil in a skillet and heat over moderate flame. Pour the Cajun-seasoned shrimp in the skillet. Broil for one minute until they are browned. Flip and then cook for two minutes.

4. Take a large-sized bowl and add the romaine lettuce to it along with tomatoes, Caesar dressing, and the parmesan cheese. Divide the entire thing between two dishes and then top with Cajun-coated shrimp.

Egg, Sausage, and Cheese Bites

Total Prep & Cooking Time: 35 minutes

Yields: Thirty-two bites

Nutrition Facts: Calories: 79 | Carbs: 1.2g | Protein: 5g | Fat: 5.9g | Fiber: 0.5g

Ingredients:

- One lb. of cooked breakfast sausage (drained and cooked)
- Three beaten eggs
- One-third cup of coconut flour
- Four oz. of softened cream cheese
- One cup of cheddar cheese (shredded)
- Half tsp. of baking powder

Method:

1. Set the oven at a temperature of 350 degrees F and keep it preheated.

2. Place a pan on the oven and put the sausage in it. Cook the breakfast sausage and drain the excess water from it. Remove it from the pan and set aside to cool slightly.

3. Take a bowl and place the cooled down sausage. Then add the cheddar cheese to the bowl. Combine them thoroughly until all the cheese clumps of cream vanish.

4. Make sure the sausage is cooled down completely before moving on to the next step. If the sausage is still hot, then it will cook the egg when added to it after this step.

5. To the sausage mixture, add the eggs, baking powder, cheese, and coconut flour.

6. Combine well to incorporate. After the ingredients are thoroughly mixed, allow them to cool down for ten minutes. The flour will continue absorbing the mixture.

7. On an adequately greased baking sheet, place the cheese bites and sausage-egg mixture. Keep them arranged in rows. Bake them for twenty minutes.

Notes: *You must chill the dough before adding in the egg mixture, as avoiding this step would lead to flat bites.*

Sheet Pan Chicken Fajitas

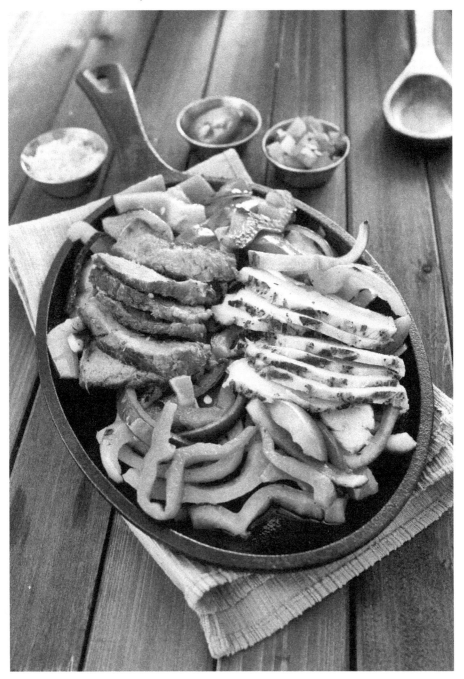

Total Prep & Cooking Time: 30 minutes

Yields: Six servings

Nutrition Facts: Calories: 357 | Carbs: 32.5g | Protein: 30.1g | Fat: 12.1g | Fiber: 6g

Ingredients:

- A quarter cup of taco seasoning
- One lime juiced
- One thinly sliced red onion
- One thinly chopped bell pepper (yellow)
- Small-sized tortillas (made of flour and warmed), optional
- Avocado
- Hot sauce
- Cilantro
- One tablespoon of olive oil
- Two pounds of chicken breasts (skinless and boneless, sliced into thin pieces)
- One bell pepper, red (chopped thinly)
- One green bell pepper (thinly chopped)

Method:

1. Take a large-sized bowl and add the lime juice, taco seasoning, and olive oil. Whisk this mixture together to form a marinade.

2. Then add the red onion, bell peppers (red, green, and yellow) and the chicken pieces to the marinade. Combine them thoroughly with a spoon. You should whisk the ingredients properly so that everything is mixed well. You can bake it at the very moment but, you can marinate for one hour before starting with the baking process to get a better taste.

3. Set the oven at a temperature of 375 degrees Fahrenheit for preheating.

4. Now take a sheet pan (preferably a rimmed one). On the sheet pan, arrange veggies and baked chicken. Bake for another twenty minutes until you cook the chicken thoroughly. If you like to have it overcooked, then broil for another three minutes.

5. After it is done, transfer them to serving plates. Garnish with hot sauce, tortillas (warmed), sour cream, avocado, and top with fresh cilantro.

6. Have it warm and enjoy it.

Chicken Shawarma Kebab

Total Prep & Cooking Time: 1 hour 10 minutes

Yields: Six servings

Nutrition Facts: Calories: 475 | Carbs: 48g | Protein: 41.6g | Fat: 13.2g | Fiber: 4.2g

Ingredients:

- Three pounds of chicken thigh (skinless and boneless)
- Two teaspoons each of
  - Cumin
  - Turmeric
  - Salt
  - Cardamom
  - Cinnamon
- One cup of yogurt (plain Greek)
- Parsley, fresh (optional)

For preparing the Tahini sauce,

- One cup of tahini (simple truth)
- Four cloves of garlic, diced
- One teaspoon of salt
- Half a cup of lemon juice
- One cup of water

Method:

1. Cut the chicken thigh into pieces of one inch each.

2. Take a bowl and place the yogurt, cardamom, cumin, turmeric, salt, and cinnamon. Add the sliced chicken pieces and then toss them properly. Combine with the help of spoon so that they can incorporate well. Cover the bowl with a lid or wrap the mouth with a paper completely and place it inside the refrigerator. Allow it to stay there for one hour.

3. Skewer the meat tightly with the help of metal skewers or soaked bamboo.

4. Keep the grill preheated to moderate heat. Place the marinated skewers on the rack and then cook the chicken thoroughly. Flip the pieces very often to ensure even cooking.

5. Take a small bowl and combine the ingredients for preparing the tahini sauce as listed above. Continue to stir the ingredients for one minute, even if they keep separating. After some time, they won't.

6. Serve the chicken with the tahini sauce and with cucumber and tomato.

One-Pan Cabbage Casserole

Total Prep & Cooking Time: 20 minutes

Yields: Six servings

Nutrition Facts: Calories: 240 | Carbs: 9g | Protein: 18.9g | Fat: 14.4g | Fiber: 1.6g

Ingredients:

- One lb. of turkey or beef (ground, drained, and browned)
- Half the head of cabbage (diced to form medium-sized chunks), approximately three cups
- Eighteen oz. of tomato sauce
- Pepper
- Salt
- One tsp. each of
  - Garlic powder
  - Chili powder
- One cup of cheese, shredded
- One small-sized onion, minced
- One can of green chilies with tomatoes

Method:

1. Turn the flame to moderate heat, place a skillet over it, and pour some oil. Add the turkey or beef to the oil and cook to make them brown. Drain off the extra grease.

2. Then add onion and stir for three to five minutes.

3. Add the tomatoes, tomato sauce, cabbage, green chilies, and the spices. Stir them well.

4. Cover the skillet and reduce the heat. Simmer for eighteen minutes and keep stirring occasionally.

5. Top the preparation with cheese and serve.

Chapter 4: One-Week Meal Plan

Here is a one-week meal plan to help you plan your days.

Monday

Breakfast – Tropical Smoothie Bowl

Lunch – Strawberry Salad

Dinner – Sheet Pan Chicken Fajitas

Snacks – Peanut Butter Balls

Tuesday

Breakfast – Banana Pancakes

Lunch – Cajun Shrimp Caesar Salad

Dinner – Zucchini Noodles and Turkey Meatballs

Snacks – Low Carb Green Smoothie

Wednesday

Breakfast – Breakfast Yogurt Parfait

Lunch – BLT Chicken Salad

Dinner – Sheet Pan Chicken Fajitas

Snacks – Peanut Butter Balls

Thursday

Breakfast – Tropical Smoothie Bowl

Lunch – Strawberry Salad

Dinner – Rosemary-Lemon Chicken

Snacks – Low Carb Green Smoothie

Friday

Breakfast – Smoked Salmon and Avocado Omelet

Lunch – BLT Chicken Salad

Dinner – Cucumber Salmon Panzanella

Snacks – Low Carb Cheesecake

Saturday

Breakfast – Breakfast Yogurt Parfait

Lunch – Mushroom and Asparagus Frittata

Dinner – Zucchini Noodles and Turkey Meatballs

Snacks – Peanut Butter Balls

Sunday

Breakfast – Tropical Smoothie Bowl

Lunch – One-Pan Cabbage Casserole

Dinner – Black Beans and Chicken Chili

Snacks – Egg, Sausage, and Cheese Bites

PART V

In this chapter, we are going to study the details of the reset diet and what recipes you can make.

Chapter 1: How to Reset Your Body?

Created by a celebrity trainer, Harley Pasternak, the body reset diet is a famous fifteen-day eating pattern that aims to jump-start weight loss. According to Pasternak, if you experience rapid loss in weight early in a diet, you will feel more motivated to stick to that diet plan. This theory is even supported by a few scientific studies (Alice A Gibson, 2017).

The body reset diet claims to help in weight loss with light exercise and low-calorie diet plans for fifteen days. The diet is divided into 3 phases of five days each. Each phase had a particular pattern of diet and exercise routine. You need to consume food five times every day, starting from the first phase, which mostly consists of smoothies and progressing to more solid foods in the second and third phases.

The three phases of the body reset diet are:

- **Phase One –** During this stage, you are required to consume only two snacks every day and drink smoothies for breakfast, lunch, and dinner. In the case of exercise, you have to walk at least ten thousand steps per day.

- **Phase Two** – During this phase, you can eat two snacks each day, consume solid food only once, and have to replace any two meals of the day with smoothies. In case of exercise, apart from walking ten thousand steps every day, on three of the days, you also have to finish five minutes of resistance training with the help of four separate exercises.

- **Phase Three** – You can consume two snacks every day, but you have to eat two low-calorie meals and replace one of your meals with a smoothie. For exercise, you are required to walk ten thousand steps. Apart from that, you also have to finish five minutes of resistance training with the help of four separate exercises each day.

After you have finished the standard fifteen-day diet requirements, you have to keep following the meal plan you followed in the third phase. However, during this time, you are allowed to have two "free meals" twice a week in which you can consume anything you want. These "free meals" are meant as a reward so that you can avoid feeling deprived. According to Pasternak, depriving yourself of a particular food continuously can result in binge eating (Nawal Alajmi, 2016).

There is no official endpoint of the diet after the first fifteen days for losing and maintaining weight. Pasternak suggests that the habits and routines formed over fifteen days should be maintained for a lifetime.

Chapter 2: Science Behind Metabolism Reset

Several people take on a "cleanse" or "detox" diet every year to lose the extra holiday weight or simply start following healthy habits. However, some fat diet plans are often a bit overwhelming. For example, it requires a tremendous amount of self-discipline to drink only juices. Moreover, even after finishing a grueling detox diet plan, you might just go back to eating foods that are bad for you because of those days of deprivation. New studies issued in the *Medicine & Science in Sports & Exercise* shows that low-calorie diets may result in binge eating, which is not the right method for lasting weight loss.

Another research conducted by the researchers at Loughborough University showed that healthy, college-aged women who followed a calorie-restricted diet consumed an extra three hundred calories at dinner as compared to the control group who consumed three standard meals. They revealed that it was because they had lower levels of peptide YY (represses appetite) and higher levels of ghrelin (makes you hungry). They are most likely to go hog wild when you are feeling ravenous, and it's finally time to eat (Nawal Alajmi K. D.-O., 2016).

Another research published in *Cognitive Neuroscience* studied the brains of chronic dieters. They revealed that there was a weaker connection between the two regions of the brain in people who had a higher percentage of body fat. They showed that they might have an increased risk of getting obese because it's harder for them to set their temptations aside (Pin-Hao Andy Chen, 2016).

A few other studies, however, also revealed that you could increase your self-control through practice. Self-control, similar to any other kind of strength, also requires time to develop. However, you can consider focusing on a diet plan that can help you "reset" instead of putting all your efforts into developing your self-control to get healthy.

A reset is considered as a new start – one that can get your metabolism and your liver in good shape. The liver is the biggest solid organ of your body, and it's mainly responsible for removing toxins that can harm your health and well-being by polluting your system. Toxins keep accumulating in your body all the time, and even though it's the liver's job to handle this, it can sometimes get behind schedule, which can result in inflammation. It causes a lot of strain on your metabolism and results in weight gain, particularly around the abdomen. The best method to alleviate this inflammation is to follow a metabolism rest diet and give your digestive system a vacation (Olivia M. Farr, 2015).

Chapter 3: Recipes for Smoothies and Salads

If you want to lose weight and you have a particular period within which you want to achieve it, then here are some recipes that are going to be helpful.

Green Smoothie

Total Prep & Cooking Time: 2 minutes

Yields: 1 serving

Nutrition Facts: Calories: 144 | Carbs: 28.2g | Protein: 3.4g | Fat: 2.9g | Fiber: 4.8g

Ingredients:

- One cup each of
  o   Almond milk
  o   Raw spinach
- One-third of a cup of strawberries
- One orange, peeled

Method:

1. Add the peeled orange, strawberries, almond milk, and raw spinach in a blender and blend everything until you get a smooth paste. You can add extra water if required to achieve the desired thickness.

2. Pour out the smoothie into a glass and serve.

Strawberry Banana Smoothie

Total Prep & Cooking Time: 5 minutes

Yields: 2 servings

Nutrition Facts: Calories: 198| Carbs: 30.8g | Protein: 5.9g | Fat: 7.1g | Fiber: 4.8g

Ingredients:

- Half a cup each of
  - Milk
  - Greek yogurt
- One banana, frozen and quartered
- Two cups of fresh strawberries, halved

Method:

1. Add the milk, Greek yogurt, banana, and strawberries into a high-powered blender and blend until you get a smooth mixture.

2. Pour the smoothie equally into two separate glasses and serve.

***Note**s:*

- *Don't add ice to the smoothie as it can make it watery very quickly. Using frozen bananas will keep your smoothie cold.*

- *As you're using bananas and strawberries, there is no need to add any artificial sweetener.*

Salmon Citrus Salad

Total Prep & Cooking Time: 20 minutes

Yields: 6 servings

Nutrition Facts: Calories: 336 | Carbs: 20g | Protein: 17g | Fat: 21g | Fiber: 5g

Ingredients:

- One pound of Citrus Salmon (slow-roasted)
- Half of an English cucumber, sliced
- One tomato (large), sliced into a quarter of an inch thick pieces
- One grapefruit, peeled and cut into segments
- Two oranges, peeled and cut into segments
- Three beets, roasted and quartered
- One avocado
- Boston lettuce leaves
- Two tablespoons of red wine vinegar
- Half of a red onion
- Flakey salt
- Aleppo pepper flakes

For the Citrus Shallot Vinaigrette,

- Five tablespoons of olive oil (extra-virgin)
- One clove of garlic, smashed
- Salt and pepper
- One and a half tablespoons of rice wine vinegar
- Two tablespoons of orange juice or fresh lemon juice

- One tablespoon of shallot, minced

Method:

For preparing the Citrus Shallot Vinaigrette:

1. Add the ingredients for the vinaigrette in a bowl and whisk them together.

2. Keep the mixture aside.

For assembling the salad,

1. Add the onions and vinegar in a small bowl and pickle them by letting them sit for about fifteen minutes.

2. In the meantime, place the lettuce leaves on the serving plate.

3. Dice the avocado in half and eliminate the pit. Then scoop the flesh and add them onto the plate. Sprinkle a dash of flakey salt and Aleppo pepper on top to season it.

4. Add the quartered beets onto the serving plate along with the grapefruit and orange segments.

5. Salt the cucumber and tomato slices lightly and add them onto the plate.

6. Then, scatter the pickled onions on top and cut the salmon into bits and add it on the plate.

7. Lastly, drizzle the Citrus Shallot Vinaigrette on top of the salad and finish off with a dash of flakey salt.

Chapter 4: Quick and Easy Breakfast and Main Course Recipes

Quinoa Salad

Total Prep & Cooking Time: 40 minutes

Yields: Eight servings

Nutrition Facts: Calories: 205 | Carbs: 25.9g | Protein: 6.1g | Fat: 9.4g | Fiber: 4.6g

Ingredients:

- One tablespoon of red wine vinegar
- One-fourth of a cup each of
  - Lemon juice (about two to three lemons)
  - Olive oil
- One cup each of
  - Quinoa (uncooked), rinsed with the help of a fine-mesh colander
  - Flat-leaf parsley (from a single large bunch), finely chopped
- Three-fourth of a cup of red onion (one small red onion), chopped
- One red bell pepper (medium-sized), chopped
- One cucumber (medium-sized), seeded and chopped
- One and a half cups of chickpeas (cooked), or One can of chickpeas (about fifteen ounces), rinsed and drained
- Two cloves of garlic, minced or pressed
- Two cups of water
- Black pepper, freshly ground
- Half a teaspoon of fine sea salt

Method:

1. Place a medium-sized saucepan over medium-high heat and add the rinsed quinoa into it along with the water. Allow the mixture to boil and then reduce the heat and simmer it. Cook for about fifteen minutes so that the quinoa has absorbed all the water. As time goes on, decrease the heat and maintain a gentle simmer. Take the saucepan away from the heat and cover it with a lid. Allow the cooked quinoa to rest for about five minutes to give it some time to increase in size.

2. Add the onions, bell pepper, cucumber, chickpeas, and parsley in a large serving bowl and mix them together. Keep the mixture aside.

3. Add the garlic, vinegar, lemon juice, olive oil, and salt in another small bowl and whisk the ingredients so that they are appropriately combined. Keep this mixture aside.

4. When the cooked quinoa has almost cooled down, transfer it to the serving bowl. Add the dressing on top and toss to combine everything together.

5. Add an extra pinch of sea salt and the black pepper to season according to your preference. Allow the salad to rest for five to ten minutes before serving it for the best results.

6. You can keep the salad in the refrigerator for up to four days. Make sure to cover it properly.

7. You can serve it at room temperature or chilled.

Notes: *Instead of cooking additional quinoa, you can use about three cups of leftover quinoa for making this salad. Moreover, you can also serve this salad with fresh greens and an additional drizzle of lemon juice and olive oil. You can also add a dollop of cashew sour cream or crumbled feta cheese as a topping.*

Herb and Goat Cheese Omelet

Total Prep & Cooking Time: 20 minutes

Yields: Two servings

Nutrition Facts: Calories: 233 | Carbs: 3.6g | Protein: 16g | Fat: 17.6g | Fiber: 1g

Ingredients:

- Half a cup each of
  - Red bell peppers (3 x quarter-inch), julienne-cut
  - Zucchini, thinly sliced
- Four large eggs
- Two teaspoons of olive oil, divided
- One-fourth of a cup of goat cheese (one ounce), crumbled
- Half a teaspoon of fresh tarragon, chopped
- One teaspoon each of
  - Fresh parsley, chopped
  - Fresh chives, chopped
- One-eighth of a teaspoon of salt
- One-fourth of a teaspoon of black pepper, freshly ground (divided)
- One tablespoon of water

Method:

1. Break the eggs into a bowl and add one tablespoon of water into it. Whisk them together and add in one-eighth of a teaspoon each of salt and ground black pepper.

2. In another small bowl, mix the goat cheese, tarragon, and parsley and keep it aside.

3. Place a nonstick skillet over medium heat and heat one teaspoon of olive oil in it. Add in the sliced zucchini, bell pepper, and the remaining one-eighth of a teaspoon of black pepper along with a dash of salt. Cook for about four minutes so that the bell pepper and zucchini get soft. Transfer the zucchini-bell pepper mixture onto a plate and cover it with a lid to keep it warm.

4. Add about half a teaspoon of oil into a skillet and add in half of the whisked egg into it. Do not stir the eggs and let the egg set slightly. Loosen the set edges of the omelet carefully with the help of a spatula. Tilt the skillet to move the uncooked part of the egg to the side. Keep following this method for about five seconds so that there is no more runny egg in the skillet. Add half of the crumbled goat cheese mixture evenly over the omelet and let it cook for another minute so that it sets.

5. Transfer the omelet onto a plate and fold it into thirds.

6. Repeat the process with the rest of the egg mixture, half a teaspoon of olive oil, and the goat cheese mixture.

7. Add the chopped chives on top of the omelets and serve with the bell pepper and zucchini mixture.

Mediterranean Cod

Total Prep & Cooking Time: 15 minutes

Yields: 4 servings

Nutrition Facts: Calories: 320 | Carbs: 31g | Protein: 35g | Fat: 8g | Fiber: 8g

Ingredients:

- One pound of spinach
- Four fillets of cod (almost one and a half pounds)
- Two zucchinis (medium-sized), chopped
- One cup of marinara sauce
- One-fourth of a teaspoon of red pepper, crushed
- Two cloves of garlic, chopped
- One tablespoon of olive oil
- Salt and pepper, according to taste
- Whole wheat roll, for serving

Method:

1. Place a ten-inch skillet on medium heat and add the marinara sauce and zucchini into it. Combine them together and let it simmer on medium heat.

2. Add the fillets of cod into the simmering sauce. Add one-fourth of a teaspoon each of salt and pepper too. Cover the skillet with a lid and let it cook for about seven minutes so that the cod gets just opaque throughout.

3. In the meantime, place a five-quart saucepot on medium heat and heat the olive oil in it. Add in the crushed red pepper and minced garlic. Stir and cook for about a minute.

4. Then, add in the spinach along with one-eighth of a teaspoon of salt. Cover the saucepot with a lid and let it cook for about five minutes, occasionally stirring so that the spinach gets wilted.

5. Add the spinach on the plates and top with the sauce and cod mixture and serve with the whole wheat roll.

Grilled Chicken and Veggies

Total Prep & Cooking Time: 35 minutes

Yields: 4 servings

Nutrition Facts: Calories: 305 | Carbs: 11g | Protein: 26g | Fat: 17g | Fiber: 3g

Ingredients:

For the marinade,

- Four cloves of garlic, crushed

- One-fourth of a cup each of
  - Fresh lemon juice
  - Olive oil
- One teaspoon each of
  - Salt
  - Smoked paprika
  - Dried oregano
- Black pepper, according to taste
- Half a teaspoon of red chili flakes

For the grilling,

- Two to three zucchinis or courgette (large), cut into thin slices
- Twelve to sixteen spears of asparagus, woody sides trimmed
- Broccoli
- Two bell peppers, seeds eliminated and cut into thin slices
- Four pieces of chicken breasts (large), skinless and de-boned

Method:

1. Preheat your griddle or grill pan.

2. Sprinkle some salt on top of the chicken breasts to season them. Keep them aside to rest while you prepare the marinade.

3. For the marinade, mix all the ingredients properly.

4. Add about half of the marinade over the vegetables and the other half over the seasoned chicken breasts. Allow the marinade to rest for a couple of minutes.

5. Place the chicken pieces on the preheated grill. Grill for about five to seven minutes on each side until they are cooked according to your preference. The time on the grill depends on the thickness of the chicken breasts.

6. Remove them from the grill and cover them using a foil. Set it aside to rest and prepare to grill the vegetables in the meantime.

7. Grill the vegetables for a few minutes until they begin to char and are crispy yet tender.

8. Remove them from the grill and transfer them onto a serving plate. Serve the veggies along with the grilled chicken and add the lemon wedges on the side for squeezing.

Notes: You can add as much or as little vegetables as you like. The vegetable amounts are given only as a guide. Moreover, feel free to replace some of them with the vegetables you like to eat.

Stuffed Peppers

Total Prep & Cooking Time: 50 minutes

Yields: 4 servings

Nutrition Facts: Calories: 438 | Carbs: 32g | Protein: 32g | Fat: 20g | Fiber: 5g

Ingredients:

For the stuffed peppers,

- One pound of ground chicken or turkey
- Four bell peppers (large) of any color
- One and a quarter of a cups of cheese, shredded
- One and a half cups of brown rice, cooked (you can use cauliflower rice or quinoa)
- One can (about fourteen ounces) of fire-roasted diced tomatoes along with its juices
- Two teaspoons of olive oil (extra-virgin)
- One teaspoon each of
  - Garlic powder
  - Ground cumin
- One tablespoon of ground chili powder
- One-fourth of a teaspoon of black pepper
- Half a teaspoon of kosher salt

For serving,

- Sour cream or Greek yogurt

- Salsa

- Freshly chopped cilantro

- Avocado, sliced

- Freshly squeezed lemon juice

Method:

1. Preheat your oven to 375 degrees Fahrenheit.

2. Take a nine by thirteen-inch baking dish and coat it lightly with a nonstick cooking spray.

3. Take the bell peppers and slice them from top to bottom into halves. Remove the membranes and the seeds. Keep the bell peppers in the baking dish with the cut-side facing upwards.

4. Place a large, nonstick skillet on medium-high heat and heat the olive oil in it. Add in the chicken, pepper, salt, garlic powder, ground cumin, and chili powder and cook for about four minutes so that the chicken is cooked through and gets brown. Break apart the chicken while it's cooking. Drain off any excess liquid and then add in the can of diced tomatoes along with the juices. Allow it to simmer for a minute.

5. Take the pan away from the heat. Add in the cooked rice along with three-fourth of a cup of the shredded cheese and stir everything together.

6. Add this filling inside the peppers and add the remaining shredded cheese as a topping.

7. Add a little amount of water into the pan containing the peppers so that it barely covers the bottom of the pan.

8. Keep it uncovered and bake it in the oven for twenty-five to thirty-five minutes so that the cheese gets melted and the peppers get soft.

9. Add any of your favorite fixings as a topping and serve hot.

Notes:

- *For preparing the stuffed peppers ahead of time, make sure to allow the rice and chicken mixture to cool down completely before filling the peppers. You can prepare the stuffed peppers before time, and then you have to cover it with a lid and keep it in the refrigerator for a maximum of twenty-four hours before baking the peppers.*

- *If you're planning to reheat the stuffed peppers, gently reheat them in your oven or microwave. If you're using a microwave for this purpose, make sure to cut the peppers into pieces to warm them evenly.*

- *You can store any leftovers in the freezer for up to three months. Alternatively, you can keep them in the refrigerator for up to four days. Allow it to thaw in the fridge overnight.*

Brussels Sprouts With Honey Mustard Chicken

Total Prep & Cooking Time: Fifty minutes

Yields: Four servings

Nutrition Facts: Calories: 360 | Carbs: 14.5g | Protein: 30.8g | Fat: 20g | Fiber: 3.7g

Ingredients:

- One and a half pounds of Brussels sprouts, divided into two halves
- Two pounds of chicken thighs, skin-on and bone-in (about four medium-sized thighs)
- Three cloves of garlic, minced
- One-fourth of a large onion, cut into slices
- One tablespoon each of
  - Honey
  - Whole-grain mustard
  - Dijon mustard
- Two tablespoons of freshly squeezed lemon juice (one lemon)
- One-fourth of a cup plus two tablespoons of olive oil (extra-virgin)
- Freshly ground black pepper
- Kosher salt
- Non-stick cooking spray

Method:

1. Preheat your oven to 425 degrees Fahrenheit.

2. Take a large baking sheet and grease it with nonstick cooking spray. Keep it aside.

3. Add the minced garlic, honey, whole-grain mustard, Dijon mustard, one tablespoon of the lemon juice, one-fourth cup of the olive oil in a medium-sized bowl and mix them together. Add the Kosher salt and black pepper to season according to your preference.

4. Dip the chicken thighs into the sauce with the help of tongs and coat both sides. Transfer the things on the baking sheet. You can get rid of any extra sauce.

5. Mix the red onion and Brussels sprouts in a medium-sized bowl and drizzle one tablespoon of lemon juice along with the remaining two tablespoons of olive oil onto it. Toss everything together until the vegetables are adequately coated.

6. Place the red onion-Brussels sprouts mixture on the baking sheet around the chicken pieces. Ensure that the chicken and vegetables are not overlapping.

7. Sprinkle a little amount of salt and pepper on the top and keep it in the oven to roast for about thirty to thirty-five minutes so that the Brussels sprouts get crispy and the chicken has an internal temperature of 165 degrees Fahrenheit and has turned golden brown.

8. Serve hot.

Quinoa Stuffed Chicken
Total Prep & Cooking Time: 50 minutes

Yields: Four servings

Nutrition Facts: Calories: 355 | Carbs: 28g | Protein: 30g | Fat: 13g | Fiber: 4g

Ingredients:

- One and a half cups of chicken broth
- Three-fourths of a cup of quinoa (any color of your choice)
- Four chicken breasts (boneless and skinless)
- One lime, zested and one tablespoon of lime juice
- One-fourth of a cup of cilantro, chipped
- One-third of a cup of unsweetened coconut, shaved or coconut chips
- One Serrano pepper, seeded and diced
- Two cloves of garlic, minced
- Half a cup of red onion, diced
- Three-fourth of a cup of bell pepper, diced
- One tablespoon of coconut oil
- One teaspoon each of
  - Salt
  - Chili powder
  - Ground cumin

Method:

1. Preheat your oven to 375 degrees Fahrenheit.

2. Take a rimmed baking sheet and line it with parchment paper.

3. Place a medium-sized saucepan over medium-high heat and add the coconut oil in it. After it has melted, add in the Serrano peppers, garlic, red onion, and bell pepper and sauté for about one to two minutes so that they soften just a bit. Make sure that the vegetables are still bright in color. Then transfer the cooked vegetables into a bowl.

4. Add the quinoa in the empty sauce pot and increase the heat to high. Pour the chicken broth in it along with half a teaspoon of salt. Close the lid of the pot and bring it to a boil, allowing the quinoa to cook for about fifteen minutes so that the surface of the quinoa develops vent holes, and the broth has absorbed completely. Take the pot away from the heat and allow it to steam for an additional five minutes.

5. In the meantime, cut a slit along the long side in each chicken breast. It will be easier with the help of a boning knife. You are making a deep pocket in each breast, having a half-inch border around the remaining three attached sides. Keep the knife parallel to the cutting board and cut through the middle of the breast and leaving the opposite side attached. Try to cut it evenly as it's challenging to cook thick uncut portions properly in the oven. After that, add salt, cumin, and chili powder on all sides of the chicken.

6. When the quinoa has turned fluffy, add in the lime juice, lime zest, shaved coconut, and sautéed vegetables and stir them in. Taste the mixture and adjust the salt as per your preference.

7. Add the confetti quinoa mixture inside the cavity of the chicken breast. Place the stuffed breasts on the baking sheet with the quinoa facing upwards. They'll look like open envelopes.

8. Bake them in the oven for about twenty minutes.

9. Serve warm.

Kale and Sweet Potato Frittata

Total Prep & Cooking Time: 30 minutes

Yields: 4 servings

Nutrition Facts: Calories: 144 | Carbs: 10g | Protein: 7g | Fat: 9g | Fiber: 2g

Ingredients:

- Three ounces of goat cheese

- Two cloves of garlic

- Half of a red onion (small)

- Two cups each of

  - Sweet potatoes

  - Firmly packed kale, chopped

- Two tablespoons of olive oil

- One cup of half-and-half

- Six large eggs

- Half a teaspoon of pepper, freshly ground

- One teaspoon of Kosher salt

Method:

1. Preheat your oven to 350 degrees Fahrenheit.

2. Add the eggs, half-and-half, salt, and black pepper in a bowl and whisk everything together.

3. Place a ten-inch ovenproof nonstick skillet over medium heat and add one tablespoon of oil in it. Sauté the sweet potatoes in the skillet for about eight to ten minutes so that they turn soft and golden brown. Transfer them onto a plate and keep warm.

4. Next, add in the remaining one tablespoon of oil and sauté the kale along with the red onions and garlic in it for about three to four minutes so that the kale gets soft and wilted. Then, add in the whisked egg mixture evenly over the vegetables and cook for an additional three minutes.

5. Add some goat cheese on the top and bake it in the oven for ten to fourteen minutes so that it sets.

Walnut, Ginger, and Pineapple Oatmeal

Total Prep & Cooking Time: 30 minutes

Yields: 4 servings

Nutrition Facts: Calories: 323 | Carbs: 61g | Protein: 6g | Fat: 8g | Fiber: 5g

Ingredients:

- Two large eggs
- Two cups each of
  - Fresh pineapple, coarsely chopped
  - Old-fashioned rolled oats
  - Whole milk
- One cup of walnuts, chopped
- Half a cup of maple syrup
- One piece of ginger
- Two teaspoons of vanilla extract
- Half a teaspoon of salt

Method:

1. Preheat your oven to 400 degrees Fahrenheit.

2. Add the ginger, walnuts, pineapple, oats, and salt in a large bowl and mix them together. Add the mixture evenly among four ten-ounce ramekins and keep them aside.

3. Whisk the eggs along with the milk, maple syrup, and vanilla extract in a medium-sized bowl. Pour one-quarter of this mixture into each ramekin containing the oat-pineapple mixture.

4. Keep the ramekins on the baking sheet and bake them in the oven for about twenty-five minutes until the oats turn light golden brown on the top and have set properly.

5. Serve with some additional maple syrup on the side.

Caprese Salad

Total Prep & Cooking Time: 15 minutes

Yields: 4 servings

Nutrition Facts: Calories: 216 | Carbs: 4g | Protein: 13g | Fat: 16g | Fiber: 1g

Ingredients:

For the salad,

- Nine basil leaves (medium-sized)
- Eight ounces of fresh whole-milk mozzarella cheese
- Two tomatoes (medium-sized)
- One-fourth of a teaspoon of black pepper, freshly ground
- Half a teaspoon of Kosher salt, or one-fourth of a teaspoon of sea salt

For the dressing,

- One teaspoon of Dijon mustard
- One tablespoon each of
  - Balsamic vinegar
  - Olive oil

Method:

1. Add the olive oil, balsamic vinegar, and Dijon mustard into a small bowl and whisk them together with the help of a small hand whisk so that you get a smooth salad dressing. Keep it aside.

2. Cut the tomatoes into thin slices and try to get ten slices in total.

3. Cut the mozzarella into nine thin slices with the help of a sharp knife.

4. Place the slices of tomatoes and mozzarella on a serving plate, alternating and overlapping one another. Then, add the basil leaves on the top.

5. Season the salad with black pepper and salt and drizzle the prepared dressing on top.

6. Serve immediately.

One-Pot Chicken Soup

Total Prep & Cooking Time: 30 minutes

Yields: 6 servings

Nutrition Facts: Calories: 201 | Carbs: 20g | Protein: 16g | Fat: 7g | Fiber: 16g

Ingredients:

- Three cups of loosely packed chopped kale (or other greens of your choice)

- Two cups of chicken, shredded

- One can of white beans (about fifteen ounces), slightly drained

- Eight cups of broth (vegetable broth or chicken broth)

- Four cloves of garlic, minced

- One cup of yellow or white onion, diced

- One tablespoon of avocado oil (skip if you are using bacon)

- One strip of uncured bacon, chopped (optional)

- Black pepper + sea salt, according to taste

Method:

1. Place a Dutch oven or a large pot over medium heat. When it gets hot, add in the oil or bacon (optional), stirring occasionally, and allow it to get hot for about a minute.

2. Then, add in the diced onion and sauté for four to five minutes, occasionally stirring so that the onions get fragrant and translucent. Add in the minced garlic next and sauté for another two to three minutes. Be careful so as not to burn the ingredients.

3. Then, add the chicken, slightly drained white beans, and broth and bring the mixture to a simmer. Cook for about ten minutes to bring out all the flavors. Taste the mixture and add salt and pepper to season according to your preference. Add in the chopped kale in the last few minutes of cooking. Cover the pot and let it cook until the kale has wilted.

4. Serve hot.

Notes: You can store any leftovers in the freezer for up to a month. Or, you can store them in the refrigerator for a maximum of three to four days. Simply reheat on the stovetop or in the microwave and eat it later.

Chocolate Pomegranate Truffles

Total Prep & Cooking Time: 10 minutes

Yields: Twelve to Fourteen truffles

Nutrition Facts: Calories: 95 | Carbs: 26g | Protein: 1g | Fat: 2g | Fiber: 3g

Ingredients:

- One-third of a cup of pomegranate arils

- Half a teaspoon each of

  o   Vanilla extract

  o   Ground cinnamon

- Half a cup of ground flax seed

- Two tablespoons of cocoa powder (unsweetened)

- About one tablespoon of water

- One and a half cups of pitted Medjool dates

- One-eighth of a teaspoon of salt

Method:

1. Add the pitted dates in a food processor and blend until it begins to form a ball. Add some water and pulse again. Add in the vanilla, cinnamon, flax seeds, cocoa powder, and salt and blend until everything is combined properly.

2. Turn off the food processor and unplug it. Add in the pomegranate arils and fold them in the mixture so that they are distributed evenly.

3. Make twelve to fourteen balls using the mixture. You can create an outer coating or topping if you want by rolling the balls in finely shredded coconut or cocoa powder.

Notes: You can store the chocolate pomegranate truffles in the fridge in an air-tight container for a maximum of three days.